Wellness a
A Guide to He

While every precaution has been taken in the preparation of this book, the publisher assumes no responsibility for errors or omissions, or for damages resulting from the use of the information contained herein.

WELLNESS AND SAFETY: A GUIDE TO HEALTH AND CARE

First edition. November 25, 2023.

ISBN: 979-8215952214

Written by imed el arbi.

Table of Contents

Empowering Wellness: A Comprehensive Guide to Health and Safe Care Embark on a journey towards optimal health and safety with this comprehensive guide that empowers you to take control of your well-being. Discover practical strategies for preventing illness, managing chronic conditions, and creating a safe and healthy environment. This invaluable resource equips you with the knowledge and tools to live a healthier, happier, and more fulfilling life.

Understanding Wellness

1.1 Introduction to Wellness

In today's fast-paced and demanding world, it is essential to prioritize our well-being. Wellness encompasses more than just the absence of illness; it is a holistic approach to living a healthy and fulfilling life. This chapter serves as an introduction to the concept of wellness and its significance in our lives. By understanding the foundations of wellness, we can begin to make informed choices that promote our overall health and safety.

1.1.1 What is wellness?

WELLNESS IS A STATE of complete physical, mental, and social well-being. It goes beyond the absence of disease and encompasses all aspects of our lives. It is a dynamic process that involves making conscious choices and taking actions that lead to a balanced and fulfilling life. Wellness is not a destination but a lifelong journey that requires continuous effort and self-reflection.

1.1.2 The Dimensions of Wellness

WELLNESS IS MULTIDIMENSIONAL and encompasses various aspects of our lives. These dimensions include:

1. Physical Wellness: Physical wellness focuses on maintaining a healthy body through regular exercise, proper nutrition, and adequate rest. It involves taking care of our physical health and addressing any medical conditions or concerns.

2. Emotional Wellness: Emotional wellness involves understanding and managing our emotions effectively. It includes developing healthy coping mechanisms, managing stress, and nurturing positive relationships.

3. Mental Wellness: Mental wellness refers to our cognitive and intellectual well-being. It involves maintaining a positive mindset, engaging in lifelong learning, and seeking help when needed.

4. Social Wellness: Social wellness emphasizes the importance of healthy relationships and connections with others. It involves effective communication, empathy, and a sense of belonging within our communities.

5. Spiritual Wellness: Spiritual wellness is about finding meaning and purpose in life. It involves exploring our values and beliefs and connecting with something greater than ourselves.

6. Occupational Wellness: Occupational wellness focuses on finding satisfaction and fulfillment in our work or chosen profession. It involves achieving a healthy work-life balance, setting goals, and pursuing personal growth.

7. Environmental Wellness: Environmental wellness emphasizes the importance of living in a safe and

sustainable environment. It involves taking care of our surroundings, minimizing our ecological footprint, and promoting a clean and healthy environment.

8. Financial Wellness: Financial wellness involves managing our finances effectively and making informed decisions about money. It includes budgeting, saving, and planning for the future.

These dimensions are interconnected and influence one another. Achieving balance in all areas of wellness is essential for overall well-being.

1.1.3 Factors Affecting Wellness

SEVERAL FACTORS CAN impact our wellness, including:

1. Lifestyle Choices: Our daily habits and choices, such as diet, exercise, sleep, and substance use, significantly impact our overall well-being.

2. Genetics: Our genetic makeup can influence our susceptibility to certain diseases and conditions. Understanding our genetic predispositions can help us make informed decisions about our health.

3. Socioeconomic Factors: Our socioeconomic status, including income, education, and access to healthcare, can affect our wellness. Disparities in these areas can lead to inequalities in health outcomes.

4. Environment: The physical and social environment in which we live plays a crucial role in our wellness. Factors such as air and water quality, community safety, and social support networks can impact our

health.

5. Stress: Chronic stress can have a detrimental effect on our well-being. Learning effective stress management techniques is essential for maintaining wellness.

6. Relationships: The quality of our relationships, both personal and professional, can significantly impact our wellness. Positive and supportive relationships contribute to our overall well-being.

1.1.4 Benefits of Wellness

PRIORITIZING WELLNESS has numerous benefits, including:

1. Improved Physical Health: Engaging in regular exercise, eating a balanced diet, and getting enough rest can improve our physical health and reduce the risk of chronic diseases.

2. Enhanced Mental Well-being: Taking care of our mental health can improve our mood, reduce stress and anxiety, and enhance our overall quality of life.

3. Increased Energy and Vitality: When we prioritize wellness, we often experience increased energy levels and a greater sense of vitality.

4. Better Resilience: Wellness practices help us build resilience, enabling us to cope with life's challenges more effectively.

5. Improved Relationships: Nurturing our well-being allows us to cultivate healthier and more fulfilling relationships with others.

6. Increased Productivity: When we are physically and

mentally well, we are more productive and able to perform at our best in various areas of life.

7. Enhanced Quality of Life: Prioritizing wellness leads to an overall improvement in our quality of life, allowing us to enjoy life to the fullest.

By understanding the foundations of wellness and the benefits it brings, we can embark on a journey towards a healthier and more fulfilling life. In the following chapters, we will explore various aspects of wellness and learn practical strategies to promote our health and safety.

1.2 Dimensions of Wellness

Wellness is a multidimensional concept that encompasses various aspects of our lives. It goes beyond the absence of illness and focuses on achieving a state of overall well-being. Understanding the different dimensions of wellness is essential for creating a balanced and fulfilling life. In this section, we will explore the various dimensions of wellness and how they contribute to our overall health and happiness.

1.2.1 Physical Wellness

PHYSICAL WELLNESS REFERS to the state of our physical health and the ability to maintain a healthy lifestyle. It involves taking care of our bodies through regular exercise, proper nutrition, and adequate rest. Engaging in physical activities not only helps us maintain a healthy weight but also improves our cardiovascular health, strengthens our muscles, and boosts our immune system. Eating a balanced diet that includes a variety of fruits, vegetables, whole grains, and lean proteins provides our bodies with the necessary nutrients to function optimally. Getting enough sleep and managing stress are also crucial for maintaining physical wellness.

1.2.2 Emotional Wellness

EMOTIONAL WELLNESS focuses on our ability to understand and manage our emotions effectively. It involves developing healthy coping mechanisms, building resilience, and nurturing positive relationships. Emotional wellness allows us to express our feelings in a healthy way, handle stress, and maintain a positive outlook on life. It also involves being aware of our own emotional needs and taking steps to meet them. Engaging in activities that bring us joy, practicing self-care, and seeking support from loved ones are essential for nurturing emotional wellness.

1.2.3 Mental Wellness

MENTAL WELLNESS ENCOMPASSES our cognitive and psychological well-being. It involves maintaining a healthy mindset, managing stress, and seeking help when needed. Mental wellness is about having a positive attitude, being resilient, and having a sense of purpose in life. Engaging in activities that challenge our minds, such as reading, puzzles, or learning new skills, can help improve mental wellness. It is also important to practice stress management techniques, such as meditation or deep breathing exercises, to maintain a healthy mental state.

1.2.4 Social Wellness

SOCIAL WELLNESS FOCUSES on our ability to build and maintain healthy relationships with others. It involves developing effective communication skills, establishing boundaries, and fostering a sense of belonging. Social wellness is about connecting with others, building a support system, and participating in social activities. It also involves being aware of the impact of our actions on others and practicing empathy and compassion. Building and maintaining healthy relationships contributes to our overall well-being and provides a sense of fulfillment and happiness.

1.2.5 Intellectual Wellness

INTELLECTUAL WELLNESS involves engaging in activities that stimulate our minds and promote lifelong learning. It is about expanding our knowledge, being curious, and seeking intellectual challenges. Intellectual wellness can be achieved through reading, attending educational workshops, or pursuing hobbies that require mental stimulation. It also involves critical thinking, problem-solving, and being open to new ideas and perspectives. Nurturing intellectual wellness not only enhances our cognitive abilities but also contributes to personal growth and self-fulfillment.

1.2.6 Occupational Wellness

OCCUPATIONAL WELLNESS refers to finding satisfaction and fulfillment in our work or chosen profession. It involves having a sense of purpose, feeling valued, and maintaining a healthy work-life balance. Occupational wellness is about finding meaning in our work, setting goals, and continuously learning and growing in our careers. It also involves managing stress and maintaining healthy relationships with colleagues. Achieving occupational wellness allows us to experience a sense of fulfillment and satisfaction in our professional lives.

1.2.7 Environmental Wellness

ENVIRONMENTAL WELLNESS focuses on our relationship with the environment and our surroundings. It involves taking care of the planet and creating a safe and healthy environment for ourselves and future generations. Environmental wellness includes practices such as recycling, conserving energy, and reducing our carbon footprint. It also involves connecting with nature, spending time outdoors, and appreciating the beauty of the natural world. Taking steps to protect and preserve the environment contributes to our overall well-being and the well-being of the planet.

1.2.8 Spiritual Wellness

SPIRITUAL WELLNESS involves finding meaning and purpose in life through a connection with something greater than ourselves. It is about exploring our beliefs, values, and ethics and aligning our actions with them. Spiritual wellness can be achieved through practices such as meditation, prayer, or engaging in activities that bring us a sense of peace and tranquility. It also involves cultivating gratitude, practicing forgiveness, and nurturing a sense of awe and wonder. Developing spiritual wellness allows us to find inner peace, experience a sense of purpose, and live in harmony with ourselves and others.

Understanding and nurturing the various dimensions of wellness is essential for achieving a balanced and fulfilling life.

Each dimension is interconnected and contributes to our overall well-being. By taking proactive steps to improve our physical, emotional, mental, social, intellectual, occupational, environmental, and spiritual wellness, we can enhance our quality of life and experience optimal health and happiness. In the following chapters, we will delve deeper into each dimension of wellness and explore practical strategies for improving and maintaining our well-being.

1.3 Factors Affecting Wellness

Wellness is a multidimensional concept that encompasses various aspects of our lives. It is influenced by a wide range of factors that can either promote or hinder our overall well-being. Understanding these factors is crucial in order to make informed decisions and take proactive steps towards improving our health and wellness.

1.3.1 Physical Factors

PHYSICAL FACTORS PLAY a significant role in determining our wellness. These include our genetic makeup, age, gender, and overall physical health. Our genetic predisposition can influence our susceptibility to certain diseases and conditions, while age and gender can affect our body's ability to function optimally. Additionally, our physical health, including any chronic conditions or disabilities, can impact our overall well-being.

Maintaining a healthy lifestyle through regular exercise, proper nutrition, and adequate sleep is essential for optimizing physical wellness. Engaging in physical activity not only helps to improve cardiovascular health and maintain a healthy weight but also boosts mood and reduces the risk of chronic diseases. A balanced diet that includes a variety of nutrient-rich foods provides the necessary fuel for our bodies to function optimally. Sufficient sleep is also crucial for physical and mental restoration.

1.3.2 Emotional and Mental Factors

OUR EMOTIONAL AND MENTAL well-being greatly influence our overall wellness. Factors such as stress, anxiety, depression, and self-esteem can significantly impact our ability to lead a fulfilling and balanced life. It is important to recognize and address these factors in order to maintain optimal wellness.

Stress, in particular, can have a profound effect on our physical and mental health. Chronic stress can lead to a weakened immune system, an increased risk of cardiovascular disease, and mental health disorders. Developing effective stress management techniques, such as mindfulness, meditation, and relaxation exercises, can help reduce the negative impact of stress on our well-being.

Building resilience is another important aspect of emotional and mental wellness. Resilience allows us to bounce back from adversity and cope with life's challenges. Developing coping mechanisms, seeking support from loved ones, and practicing self-care are all essential to building resilience and maintaining emotional well-being.

1.3.3 Social Factors

OUR SOCIAL CONNECTIONS and relationships have a significant impact on our wellness. Positive and supportive relationships can provide a sense of belonging, emotional support, and a network of resources. On the other hand, social isolation and unhealthy relationships can negatively affect our mental and physical health.

Maintaining healthy relationships involves effective communication, setting boundaries, and resolving conflicts in a constructive manner. Building and nurturing relationships that are based on trust, respect, and mutual support can greatly contribute to our overall well-being.

1.3.4 Environmental Factors

THE ENVIRONMENT IN which we live, work, and play can have a profound impact on our wellness. Factors such as air and water quality, access to green spaces, and exposure to toxins can all influence our physical and mental health.

Creating a safe and healthy environment involves taking steps to minimize exposure to environmental hazards. This can include ensuring proper ventilation in our homes, using natural and non-toxic cleaning products, and being mindful of our consumption and waste habits. Additionally, spending time in nature and engaging in outdoor activities can have a positive impact on our well-being.

1.3.5 Economic Factors

ECONOMIC FACTORS CAN also affect our wellness. Financial stability and access to resources can impact our ability to meet our basic needs, access healthcare, and engage in activities that promote well-being. Financial stress and insecurity can contribute to mental health issues and hinder our ability to lead a healthy lifestyle.

Taking steps towards financial wellness, such as budgeting, saving, and seeking financial advice when needed, can help alleviate financial stress and promote overall well-being.

1.3.6 Cultural Factors

CULTURAL FACTORS, INCLUDING our beliefs, values, and traditions, can influence our wellness. Cultural norms and expectations can shape our behaviors and attitudes towards health and well-being. It is important to recognize and respect the diversity of cultural practices and beliefs when considering wellness strategies.

Understanding and embracing cultural diversity can enhance our overall wellness by promoting inclusivity, acceptance, and a sense of belonging.

In conclusion, wellness is influenced by a multitude of factors, including physical, emotional, social, environmental, economic, and cultural aspects of our lives. By recognizing and addressing these factors, we can take proactive steps towards improving our overall well-being. Empowering ourselves with knowledge and adopting healthy lifestyle habits can lead to a happier, healthier, and more fulfilling life.

1.4 Benefits of Wellness

Wellness is not just the absence of illness; it is a state of complete physical, mental, and social well-being. When we prioritize our wellness, we reap numerous benefits that enhance our overall quality of life. In this section, we will explore the various advantages of embracing a wellness-focused lifestyle.

1.4.1 Physical Well-Being

ONE OF THE PRIMARY benefits of wellness is improved physical health. By adopting healthy habits such as regular exercise, balanced nutrition, and adequate sleep, we can enhance our physical well-being. Engaging in physical activity helps to strengthen our muscles, improve cardiovascular health, and boost our immune system. It also reduces the risk of chronic diseases such as heart disease, diabetes, and certain types of cancer.

A well-balanced diet provides our bodies with the necessary nutrients to function optimally. It supports healthy growth and development, improves digestion, and helps maintain a healthy weight. Additionally, getting enough sleep allows our bodies to rest and rejuvenate, promoting better overall health and vitality.

1.4.2 Mental and emotional well-being

WELLNESS ALSO ENCOMPASSES mental and emotional well-being. Taking care of our mental health is crucial for maintaining a balanced and fulfilling life. When we prioritize our mental well-being, we experience reduced stress levels, improved mood, and increased resilience.

Engaging in stress management techniques, such as meditation, deep breathing exercises, and mindfulness, can help us cope with the challenges of daily life. These practices promote relaxation, reduce anxiety, and improve our ability to handle stress.

Building resilience is another important aspect of mental and emotional well-being. Resilience allows us to bounce back from setbacks, adapt to change, and maintain a positive outlook. By developing resilience, we can navigate life's challenges with greater ease and maintain a sense of well-being.

1.4.3 Improved Relationships

WHEN WE PRIORITIZE our wellness, we also enhance our relationships with others. By taking care of our physical and mental health, we are better equipped to engage in meaningful connections and build strong relationships.

Good communication skills are essential for healthy relationships. When we prioritize our wellness, we are more likely to have the energy and mental clarity to effectively communicate with others. This leads to improved understanding, reduced conflicts, and stronger connections.

Additionally, when we prioritize our own well-being, we set a positive example for those around us. By taking care of ourselves, we inspire others to do the same, creating a ripple effect of wellness within our communities and relationships.

1.4.4 Increased Productivity and Performance

PRIORITIZING WELLNESS can also have a positive impact on our productivity and performance in various areas of life. When we take care of our physical health through regular exercise and proper nutrition, we experience increased energy levels and improved cognitive function. This, in turn, enhances our ability to focus, concentrate, and perform at our best in work, school, and other activities.

Furthermore, when we prioritize our mental and emotional well-being, we are better equipped to handle stress and manage our emotions effectively. This allows us to approach tasks with a clear and focused mind, leading to increased productivity and better overall performance.

1.4.5 Enhanced Quality of Life

ULTIMATELY, THE BENEFITS of wellness culminate in an enhanced quality of life. When we prioritize our well-being, we experience greater overall satisfaction and fulfillment. We are more likely to engage in activities that bring us joy and fulfillment, pursue our passions, and maintain a positive outlook on life.

By taking care of our physical, mental, and emotional health, we can enjoy a higher level of well-being and happiness. We are better equipped to handle life's challenges, maintain positive relationships, and live a life that aligns with our values and aspirations.

1.4.6 Longevity and Aging Well

ANOTHER SIGNIFICANT benefit of wellness is its impact on longevity and aging well. By adopting healthy lifestyle habits and prioritizing our well-being, we can increase our chances of living a longer and healthier life. Regular exercise, a balanced diet, and stress management techniques can help prevent age-related diseases and maintain physical and cognitive function as we age.

Furthermore, by taking care of our mental and emotional well-being, we can promote healthy aging and maintain a positive outlook on life. Building resilience and seeking support when needed can help us navigate the challenges that come with aging and maintain a high quality of life.

In conclusion, embracing wellness brings numerous benefits that enhance our physical, mental, and emotional well-being. By prioritizing our wellness, we can experience improved physical health, enhanced relationships, increased productivity, and an overall higher quality of life. Investing in our well-being is a lifelong journey that empowers us to live our best lives and thrive in all aspects of life.

Preventing Illness

2.1 Importance of Prevention

Prevention is the cornerstone of maintaining good health and well-being. By taking proactive measures to prevent illness and injury, we can significantly reduce the risk of developing chronic conditions and improve our overall quality of life. Prevention encompasses a wide range of strategies, from adopting healthy lifestyle habits to receiving regular screenings and immunizations. In this section, we will explore the importance of prevention and how it can positively impact our health.

2.1.1 Promoting Longevity

PREVENTION PLAYS A crucial role in promoting longevity and ensuring a higher quality of life as we age. By adopting healthy lifestyle habits and engaging in preventive measures, we can reduce the risk of developing chronic diseases such as heart disease, diabetes, and certain types of cancer. These conditions are often preventable through lifestyle modifications such as maintaining a balanced diet, engaging in regular physical activity, and avoiding tobacco and excessive alcohol consumption.

2.1.2 Cost-Effectiveness

PREVENTION IS NOT ONLY beneficial for our health but also for our wallets. Investing in preventive measures can save us significant healthcare costs in the long run. By preventing the onset of chronic conditions, we can avoid expensive medical treatments, hospitalizations, and medications. Additionally, preventive measures such as vaccinations and screenings are often more cost-effective than treating advanced stages of diseases.

2.1.3 Enhancing Quality of Life

PREVENTION NOT ONLY helps us avoid illness but also enhances our overall quality of life. By adopting healthy lifestyle habits, such as eating a nutritious diet and engaging in regular exercise, we can experience increased energy levels, improved mental well-being, and better sleep patterns. Preventive measures also allow us to maintain our independence and engage in activities we enjoy without the limitations imposed by chronic conditions.

2.1.4 Empowering Individuals

PREVENTION EMPOWERS individuals to take an active role in their own health and well-being. By educating ourselves about preventive measures and making informed choices, we can have a significant impact on our overall health outcomes. Taking responsibility for our health includes understanding the importance of preventive screenings, immunizations, and regular check-ups. By actively participating in our healthcare, we can detect potential health issues early on and take appropriate action.

2.1.5 Reducing the Burden on Healthcare Systems

PREVENTION PLAYS A vital role in reducing the burden on healthcare systems. By preventing the onset of chronic conditions, we can alleviate the strain on healthcare resources, including hospitals, clinics, and medical professionals. By focusing on prevention, we can shift the healthcare paradigm from a reactive approach to a proactive one, ultimately leading to more efficient and sustainable healthcare systems.

2.1.6 Creating Healthy Communities

PREVENTION EXTENDS beyond individual health and has a broader impact on communities. By promoting preventive measures, we can create healthier communities that prioritize well-being and safety. Healthy communities are characterized by access to nutritious food, safe environments, and opportunities for physical activity. By working together to promote prevention, we can create a supportive environment that fosters the health and well-being of all community members.

2.1.7 Empowering Future Generations

PREVENTION IS NOT ONLY important for our own health but also for the well-being of future generations. By adopting healthy lifestyle habits and promoting preventive measures, we can set a positive example for our children and grandchildren. Instilling the value of prevention at an early age can help create a culture of health and well-being that extends beyond our own lifetimes.

2.1.8 Addressing Health Disparities

PREVENTION IS A POWERFUL tool for addressing health disparities and promoting health equity. By focusing on prevention, we can ensure that all individuals, regardless of their socioeconomic status or background, have access to the resources and information needed to maintain good health. Preventive measures such as vaccinations and screenings can help bridge the gap in healthcare access and reduce disparities in health outcomes.

In conclusion, prevention is a fundamental aspect of maintaining good health and well-being. By prioritizing prevention, we can promote longevity, enhance our quality of life, and reduce the burden on healthcare systems. Prevention empowers individuals to take an active role in their own health and creates healthier communities for future generations. By investing in prevention, we can pave the way for a healthier, happier, and more fulfilling life.

2.2 Healthy Lifestyle Habits

I n order to maintain good health and prevent illness, it is essential to adopt healthy lifestyle habits. These habits not only contribute to physical well-being but also have a positive impact on mental and emotional health. By making small changes to your daily routine, you can significantly improve your overall well-being and reduce the risk of developing chronic conditions.

2.2.1 Balanced Diet

A BALANCED DIET IS the foundation of a healthy lifestyle. It provides the necessary nutrients, vitamins, and minerals that the body needs to function optimally. Aim to include a variety of fruits, vegetables, whole grains, lean proteins, and healthy fats in your diet. Avoid processed foods, sugary snacks, and excessive consumption of salt and saturated fats.

2.2.2 Regular Physical Activity

REGULAR PHYSICAL ACTIVITY is crucial for maintaining a healthy weight, improving cardiovascular health, and boosting mood and energy levels. Aim for at least 150 minutes of moderate-intensity aerobic activity or 75 minutes of vigorous-intensity aerobic activity per week. Additionally, incorporate strength training exercises at least twice a week to build and maintain muscle mass.

2.2.3 Adequate Sleep

SLEEP PLAYS A VITAL role in overall health and well-being. It is during sleep that the body repairs and rejuvenates itself. Aim for 7-9 hours of quality sleep each night. Establish a regular sleep schedule, create a relaxing bedtime routine, and ensure your sleep environment is comfortable and conducive to restful sleep.

2.2.4 Stress Management

STRESS CAN HAVE A DETRIMENTAL effect on both physical and mental health. It is important to develop effective stress management techniques to reduce its impact. Engage in activities that help you relax and unwind, such as meditation, deep breathing exercises, yoga, or engaging in hobbies. Prioritize self-care and make time for activities that bring you joy and peace.

2.2.5 Limit Alcohol and Tobacco Use

EXCESSIVE ALCOHOL CONSUMPTION and tobacco use can have serious health consequences. Limit your alcohol intake to moderate levels, which is defined as up to one drink per day for women and up to two drinks per day for men. If you smoke, seek support and resources to quit smoking. Avoid exposure to secondhand smoke as well.

2.2.6 Hydration

PROPER HYDRATION IS essential for maintaining optimal bodily functions. Aim to drink at least 8 cups (64 ounces) of water per day. Adjust your fluid intake based on your activity level, climate, and individual needs. Avoid excessive consumption of sugary beverages and opt for water as your primary source of hydration.

2.2.7 Regular health check-ups

REGULAR HEALTH CHECK-ups are essential for the early detection and prevention of potential health issues. Schedule routine visits with your healthcare provider to monitor your overall health, discuss any concerns or symptoms, and receive appropriate screenings and vaccinations. Stay up-to-date with recommended immunizations to protect yourself and others from preventable diseases.

2.2.8 Mindful Technology Use

IN TODAY'S DIGITAL age, it is important to be mindful of our technology use. Excessive screen time can negatively impact sleep, mental health, and social interactions. Set boundaries for screen time and prioritize face-to-face interactions. Take breaks from screens, engage in physical activities, and spend time in nature to promote overall well-being.

2.2.9 Healthy Relationships

HEALTHY RELATIONSHIPS contribute to overall well-being and happiness. Cultivate positive relationships with family, friends, and colleagues. Practice effective communication, active listening, and empathy. Set boundaries and prioritize self-care within relationships. Seek support and professional help if needed to navigate challenging relationships or situations.

2.2.10 Positive Mindset

A POSITIVE MINDSET can have a profound impact on overall well-being. Cultivate gratitude, practice self-compassion, and focus on the present moment. Surround yourself with positive influences, and engage in activities that bring you joy and fulfillment. Develop a growth mindset and embrace challenges as opportunities for personal growth and learning.

By incorporating these healthy lifestyle habits into your daily routine, you can significantly improve your overall well-being and reduce the risk of developing chronic conditions. Remember, small changes can lead to big results. Take control of your health and empower yourself to live a life of wellness and safety.

2.3 Immunizations and Vaccinations

Immunizations and vaccinations play a crucial role in preventing the spread of infectious diseases and protecting individuals from potentially harmful illnesses. By stimulating the immune system to produce antibodies, vaccines help the body recognize and fight off specific pathogens, reducing the risk of infection and its associated complications. In this section, we will explore the importance of immunizations and vaccinations, the types of vaccines available, and their impact on public health.

2.3.1 Understanding Immunizations

IMMUNIZATIONS ARE A vital component of preventive healthcare, as they provide protection against a wide range of infectious diseases. Vaccines contain weakened or inactivated forms of the disease-causing microorganism or specific parts of it, such as proteins or sugars. When administered, vaccines stimulate the immune system to produce an immune response, including the production of antibodies. These antibodies help the body recognize and destroy the pathogen if it is encountered in the future.

2.3.2 Types of Vaccines

THERE ARE SEVERAL TYPES of vaccines available, each designed to target specific diseases and provide immunity. Some common types of vaccines include:

1. **Inactivated Vaccines**: These vaccines contain killed or inactivated forms of the pathogen. Examples include the inactivated polio vaccine and the hepatitis A vaccine.
2. **Live Attenuated Vaccines**: Live attenuated vaccines contain weakened forms of the pathogen. They closely resemble a natural infection, stimulating a strong immune response. Examples include the measles, mumps, and rubella (MMR) vaccine and the oral polio vaccine.
3. **Subunit, Recombinant, and Conjugate Vaccines**: These vaccines contain specific parts of the pathogen, such as proteins or sugars. They are often used when the whole pathogen may be too dangerous to include in the vaccine. Examples include the hepatitis B vaccine and the human papillomavirus (HPV) vaccine.
4. **Toxoid Vaccines**: Toxoid vaccines target diseases caused by toxins produced by bacteria. These vaccines contain inactivated toxins that stimulate the production of antibodies. Examples include the tetanus and diphtheria vaccines.

2.3.3 Benefits of Immunizations

IMMUNIZATIONS OFFER numerous benefits to individuals and communities, including:

1. **Disease Prevention**: Vaccines are highly effective in preventing the spread of infectious diseases. By reducing the number of

susceptible individuals, vaccines help create herd immunity, protecting those who cannot be vaccinated, such as infants, pregnant women, and individuals with weakened immune systems.

2. **Reduced Disease Severity**: Even if a vaccinated individual contracts a disease, the symptoms are often milder compared to those of those who are unvaccinated. Vaccines can help prevent severe complications, hospitalizations, and even death.

3. **Eradication and Control of Diseases**: Vaccines have played a crucial role in eradicating or significantly reducing the incidence of several diseases worldwide. Diseases such as smallpox and polio have been successfully eliminated or brought under control through widespread vaccination efforts.

4. **Cost-Effectiveness**: Immunizations are a cost-effective public health intervention. The cost of vaccinating individuals against a disease is often significantly lower than the cost of treating the disease and its complications.

5. **Global Health Impact**: Vaccines have the potential to improve global health by reducing the burden of infectious diseases, particularly in low-income countries where access to healthcare resources may be limited.

2.3.4 Vaccine Safety

VACCINES UNDERGO RIGOROUS testing and monitoring to ensure their safety and efficacy. Before a vaccine is approved for use, it goes through multiple stages of clinical trials to assess its safety, effectiveness, and potential side effects. Regulatory agencies, such as the Food and Drug Administration (FDA) in the United States, carefully review the data from these trials before granting approval.

Common side effects of vaccines are generally mild and temporary, such as soreness at the injection site, low-grade fever, or fatigue. Serious side effects are rare but can occur. Vaccine safety monitoring systems continuously monitor the safety of vaccines after they are licensed and in use. These systems help identify and investigate any potential safety concerns.

It is important to note that the benefits of vaccination far outweigh the risks. The vast majority of individuals who receive vaccines experience no adverse effects and gain significant protection against infectious diseases.

2.3.5 Vaccine Recommendations and Schedules

VACCINE RECOMMENDATIONS and schedules may vary depending on factors such as age, health condition, occupation, and travel plans. National and international health organizations, such as the Centers for Disease Control and Prevention (CDC) and the World Health Organization (WHO), provide guidelines on recommended vaccines for different populations.

Children typically receive a series of vaccines starting in infancy to protect against diseases such as measles, mumps, rubella, polio, hepatitis, and influenza. Adolescents and adults may require additional vaccines, such as the HPV vaccine, meningococcal vaccine, or tetanus booster.

It is important to consult with healthcare professionals or refer to official guidelines to ensure that you and your loved ones are up to date with the recommended vaccines.

2.3.6 Vaccine Hesitancy and Misinformation

VACCINE HESITANCY, the reluctance or refusal to vaccinate despite the availability of vaccines, is a growing concern. Misinformation and misconceptions about vaccines can contribute to vaccine hesitancy. It is essential to rely on credible sources of information, such as healthcare professionals and reputable organizations, to make informed decisions about vaccination.

Public health campaigns and educational initiatives play a crucial role in addressing vaccine hesitancy and promoting accurate information about vaccines. By providing clear and evidence-based information, healthcare professionals can help individuals make informed decisions and understand the importance of immunizations in protecting their health and the health of their communities.

Conclusion

IMMUNIZATIONS AND VACCINATIONS are powerful tools for preventing the spread of infectious diseases and safeguarding individual and public health. By understanding the importance of immunizations, the different types of vaccines available, and the benefits they offer, individuals can make informed decisions about their own health and contribute to the well-being of their communities. Stay up-to-date with recommended vaccines and consult with healthcare professionals to ensure you and your loved ones are protected against vaccine-preventable diseases.

2.4 Screenings and Early Detection

Regular screenings and early detection play a crucial role in maintaining good health and preventing serious illnesses. By identifying potential health issues at an early stage, individuals have a better chance of successful treatment and improved outcomes. In this section, we will explore the importance of screenings, the different types of screenings available, and how they can contribute to overall wellness.

2.4.1 Understanding screenings

SCREENINGS ARE MEDICAL tests or examinations that are performed to detect the presence of a particular disease or condition before any symptoms appear. These tests are typically quick, non-invasive, and can be done in a variety of healthcare settings, including hospitals, clinics, and specialized screening centers. The goal of screenings is to identify potential health problems early on, when they are most treatable.

2.4.2 Types of Screenings

THERE ARE VARIOUS TYPES of screenings available, each targeting specific diseases or conditions. Some common screenings include the following:

2.4.2.1 Cancer Screenings

CANCER SCREENINGS ARE designed to detect the presence of cancer or precancerous cells in the body. Examples of cancer screenings include mammograms for breast cancer, Pap smears for cervical cancer, colonoscopies for colorectal cancer, and prostate-specific antigen (PSA) tests for prostate cancer. These screenings are essential for early detection and can significantly increase the chances of successful treatment.

2.4.2.2 Cardiovascular Screenings

CARDIOVASCULAR SCREENINGS are aimed at assessing an individual's risk for heart disease and stroke. These screenings may include blood pressure measurements, cholesterol level checks, electrocardiograms (ECGs), and stress tests. By identifying risk factors early on, individuals can take steps to manage their cardiovascular health and reduce the likelihood of developing serious heart-related conditions.

2.4.2.3 Diabetes Screenings

DIABETES SCREENINGS are used to identify individuals at risk for developing diabetes or those who may already have the condition but are unaware of it. These screenings typically involve blood tests to measure blood glucose levels. Early detection of diabetes allows for timely intervention and the implementation of lifestyle changes or medical treatments to manage the condition effectively.

2.4.2.4 Vision and Hearing Screenings

VISION AND HEARING screenings are essential for maintaining optimal sensory health. These screenings can detect vision problems such as nearsightedness, farsightedness, and astigmatism, as well as identify hearing loss or other auditory issues. Early detection of these conditions can lead to appropriate interventions, such as corrective lenses or hearing aids, to improve the overall quality of life.

2.4.2.5 Bone Density Screenings

BONE DENSITY SCREENINGS, also known as dual-energy X-ray absorptiometry (DXA) scans, are used to assess bone health and detect osteoporosis, or low bone density. These screenings are particularly important for postmenopausal women and older adults, as they are at a higher risk of developing osteoporosis. Early detection allows for the implementation of preventive measures and appropriate treatments to reduce the risk of fractures and maintain bone health.

2.4.3 Benefits of Screenings

REGULAR SCREENINGS offer several benefits for individuals of all ages. Some of the key advantages include:

2.4.3.1 Early Detection and Treatment

ONE OF THE PRIMARY benefits of screenings is the early detection of diseases or conditions. By identifying potential health issues before symptoms appear, individuals have a better chance of successful treatment and improved outcomes. Early intervention can often prevent the progression of a disease or condition, leading to a better quality of life.

2.4.3.2 Prevention and Risk Reduction

SCREENINGS CAN HELP identify risk factors for certain diseases or conditions, allowing individuals to take proactive steps to reduce their risk. For example, if a screening reveals high cholesterol levels, individuals can make lifestyle changes, such as adopting a healthier diet and increasing physical activity, to lower their risk of heart disease.

2.4.3.3 Peace of Mind

REGULAR SCREENINGS can provide individuals with peace of mind, knowing that they are taking proactive steps to monitor their health. By staying on top of their health status, individuals can feel more confident and empowered in their overall well-being.

2.4.4 Screening Guidelines

IT IS IMPORTANT TO follow recommended screening guidelines based on age, gender, and individual risk factors.

These guidelines are developed by medical experts and organizations to ensure that individuals receive the appropriate screenings at the right time. It is essential to consult with a healthcare professional to determine which screenings are necessary for your specific circumstances.

2.4.5 Conclusion

SCREENINGS AND EARLY detection are vital components of maintaining good health and preventing serious illnesses. By staying proactive and following recommended guidelines, individuals can take control of their well-being and increase their chances of early intervention and successful treatment. Regular screenings, along with healthy lifestyle habits and preventive measures, contribute to overall wellness and a higher quality of life.

MANAGING CHRONIC CONDITIONS

3.1 Understanding Chronic Conditions

Chronic conditions are long-term health conditions that require ongoing management and care. Unlike acute illnesses, which are short-lived and often resolve on their own, chronic conditions persist for an extended period and may even last a lifetime. These conditions can significantly impact a person's quality of life and require careful attention and management.

3.1.1 What are chronic conditions?

CHRONIC CONDITIONS encompass a wide range of health issues that affect various body systems. Some common examples include diabetes, heart disease, asthma, arthritis, and chronic pain. These conditions can be caused by a combination of genetic, environmental, and lifestyle factors. While some chronic conditions are preventable, others may develop due to factors beyond an individual's control.

3.1.2 The Impact of Chronic Conditions

LIVING WITH A CHRONIC condition can have a profound impact on a person's physical, emotional, and social well-being. The symptoms and limitations associated with these conditions can affect daily activities, work, relationships, and the overall quality of life. Chronic conditions often require ongoing medical treatment, regular monitoring, and lifestyle modifications to manage symptoms and prevent complications.

3.1.3 Common Types of Chronic Conditions

THERE ARE NUMEROUS chronic conditions that individuals may face throughout their lives. Some of the most prevalent chronic conditions include:

1. Diabetes is a condition characterized by high blood sugar levels due to the body's inability to produce or effectively use insulin. Diabetes can lead to serious complications if not properly managed.
2. Heart disease is a broad term that encompasses various conditions affecting the heart, including coronary artery disease, heart failure, and arrhythmias. Heart disease is a leading cause of death worldwide.
3. Asthma is a chronic respiratory condition that causes inflammation and narrowing of the airways, leading to breathing difficulties. Asthma symptoms can range from mild to severe and may require ongoing medication and management.
4. Arthritis is a group of conditions that cause inflammation and stiffness in the joints. Arthritis can result in pain, swelling, and reduced mobility, affecting daily activities and overall quality of life.
5. Chronic pain: persistent pain that lasts for more than

three months and can be caused by various factors, including injury, nerve damage, or underlying health conditions. Chronic pain can have a significant impact on a person's physical and emotional well-being.

3.1.4 Causes and Risk Factors

THE CAUSES OF CHRONIC conditions can vary depending on the specific condition. Some chronic conditions, such as type 2 diabetes and heart disease, may be influenced by lifestyle factors such as poor diet, lack of physical activity, smoking, and excessive alcohol consumption. Other chronic conditions, such as autoimmune diseases, may have a genetic or environmental component.

Certain risk factors can increase the likelihood of developing chronic conditions. These risk factors include:

- Age: The risk of developing chronic conditions tends to increase with age.

- Family History: Having a family history of a particular chronic condition can increase the risk of developing the same condition.

- Lifestyle Factors: Unhealthy lifestyle habits, such as a sedentary lifestyle, poor diet, smoking, and excessive alcohol consumption, can contribute to the development of chronic conditions.

- Environmental Factors: Exposure to certain environmental factors, such as air pollution or toxins, can increase the risk of developing chronic conditions.

3.1.5 Diagnosis and Management

DIAGNOSING A CHRONIC condition typically involves a combination of a medical history, physical examinations, laboratory tests, and imaging studies. Once diagnosed, the management of chronic conditions focuses on controlling symptoms, preventing complications, and improving overall well-being.

Treatment options for chronic conditions may include the following:

- Medications: Depending on the specific condition, medications may be prescribed to manage symptoms, control inflammation, regulate blood sugar levels, or prevent complications.

- Lifestyle Modifications: Adopting healthy lifestyle habits, such as regular exercise, a balanced diet, stress management, and adequate sleep, can play a crucial role in managing chronic conditions.

- Self-Management Strategies: Learning self-care techniques, such as monitoring symptoms, adhering to medication regimens, and making informed decisions about health, can empower individuals to take an active role in managing their condition.

- Support and Resources: Support groups, educational programs, and healthcare professionals can provide valuable guidance, information, and emotional support for individuals living with chronic conditions.

3.1.6 Living Well with Chronic Conditions

WHILE LIVING WITH A chronic condition can present challenges, it is possible to lead a fulfilling and meaningful life. By actively managing their condition and making positive lifestyle choices, individuals can improve their overall well-being and reduce the impact of their chronic condition on their daily lives.

Some strategies for living well with chronic conditions include the following:

- Education and Knowledge: Understanding the condition, its symptoms, and treatment options can empower individuals to make informed decisions about their health and actively participate in their care.

- Self-Care: Engaging in self-care activities, such as regular exercise, healthy eating, stress management, and adequate sleep, can help individuals better manage their symptoms and improve their overall well-being.

- Emotional Support: Seeking emotional support from friends, family, support groups, or mental health professionals can provide individuals with the necessary support and understanding to cope with the emotional challenges of living with a chronic condition.

• Goal Setting: Setting realistic goals and focusing on small, achievable steps can help individuals stay motivated and maintain a positive outlook on their journey towards managing their chronic condition.

• Regular Check-ups: Regular medical check-ups and monitoring can help individuals track their progress, identify any changes or complications, and make necessary adjustments to their treatment plan.

By understanding chronic conditions, their causes, and management strategies, individuals can take proactive steps towards living a healthier and more fulfilling life. With the right knowledge, support, and resources, individuals can effectively manage their chronic conditions and optimize their overall well-being.

3.2 Treatment Options

When it comes to managing chronic conditions, there are various treatment options available that can help individuals effectively control their symptoms and improve their overall quality of life. Treatment plans are often tailored to the specific condition and individual needs and may involve a combination of medical interventions, lifestyle modifications, and self-management strategies. In this section, we will explore some common treatment options for chronic conditions and discuss how they can be incorporated into a comprehensive care plan.

3.2.1 Medications

MEDICATIONS PLAY A crucial role in the management of many chronic conditions. They can help alleviate symptoms, slow down disease progression, and improve overall health outcomes. Depending on the condition, different types of medications may be prescribed. For example, individuals with diabetes may require insulin or oral medications to regulate blood sugar levels, while those with hypertension may be prescribed antihypertensive drugs to control blood pressure. It is important to follow the prescribed medication regimen and communicate any concerns or side effects to your healthcare provider.

3.2.2 Physical Therapy

PHYSICAL THERAPY IS a non-invasive treatment option that focuses on improving mobility, strength, and function. It is often recommended for individuals with musculoskeletal conditions, such as arthritis or back pain, as well as those recovering from injuries or surgeries. Physical therapists use a variety of techniques, including exercises, manual therapy, and modalities such as heat or cold therapy, to help individuals regain their physical abilities and reduce pain. They also provide education on proper body mechanics and ergonomics to prevent further injuries.

3.2.3 Rehabilitation Programs

REHABILITATION PROGRAMS are designed to help individuals recover and regain independence after a major health event, such as a stroke or heart attack. These programs typically involve a multidisciplinary approach, with healthcare professionals from various disciplines working together to address the physical, cognitive, and emotional aspects of recovery. Rehabilitation may include physical therapy, occupational therapy, speech therapy, and psychological support. The goal is to optimize function and improve overall well-being.

3.2.4 Surgical Interventions

IN SOME CASES, SURGICAL interventions may be necessary to treat or manage chronic conditions. Surgery can range from minimally invasive procedures, such as arthroscopy for joint conditions, to more complex surgeries, such as organ transplants. Surgical interventions are typically considered when other treatment options have been exhausted or when there is a significant risk to the individual's health. It is important to have a thorough discussion with your healthcare provider to understand the risks, benefits, and expected outcomes of any surgical procedure.

3.2.5 Complementary and Alternative Therapies

COMPLEMENTARY AND ALTERNATIVE therapies are non-conventional treatment options that can be used alongside traditional medical interventions. These therapies aim to promote holistic well-being and may include practices such as acupuncture, chiropractic care, herbal medicine, and mindfulness-based techniques. While the evidence for the effectiveness of these therapies varies, some individuals find them beneficial for managing their symptoms and improving their overall quality of life. It is important to consult with a qualified practitioner and inform your healthcare provider about any complementary or alternative therapies you are considering.

3.2.6 Assistive Devices and Adaptive Equipment

FOR INDIVIDUALS WITH chronic conditions that affect their mobility or daily functioning, assistive devices and adaptive equipment can greatly enhance their independence and quality of life. These devices can range from simple aids, such as canes or walkers, to more complex equipment, such as wheelchairs or prosthetics. Occupational therapists and physical therapists can assess an individual's needs and recommend appropriate assistive devices or modifications to their environment to facilitate their daily activities.

3.2.7 Lifestyle Modifications

IN ADDITION TO MEDICAL interventions, lifestyle modifications play a crucial role in managing chronic conditions. These modifications may include adopting a healthy diet, engaging in regular physical activity, managing stress, getting adequate sleep, and avoiding harmful habits such as smoking or excessive alcohol consumption. Lifestyle modifications can help improve overall health, reduce symptoms, and prevent complications associated with chronic conditions. It is important to work with your healthcare provider or a registered dietitian to develop a personalized plan that suits your specific needs and goals.

3.2.8 Supportive Therapies

LIVING WITH A CHRONIC condition can be challenging, both physically and emotionally. Supportive therapies, such as counseling, support groups, and mindfulness-based practices, can provide individuals with the tools and support they need to cope with the emotional and psychological aspects of their condition. These therapies can help individuals develop resilience, manage stress, and improve their overall well-being.

It is important to seek out appropriate resources and support networks to ensure a comprehensive approach to managing chronic conditions.

In conclusion, there are various treatment options available for managing chronic conditions. These options range from medications and physical therapy to surgical interventions and lifestyle modifications. It is important for individuals to work closely with their healthcare providers to develop a comprehensive treatment plan that addresses their specific needs and goals. By actively participating in their own care and making informed decisions, individuals can effectively manage their chronic conditions and improve their overall well-being.

3.3 Self-Management Strategies

Self-management is a crucial aspect of managing chronic conditions and maintaining overall wellness. It involves taking an active role in your own health and making informed decisions to improve your quality of life. By implementing self-management strategies, you can effectively manage your condition, reduce symptoms, and prevent complications. In this section, we will explore various self-management strategies that can empower you to take control of your health and well-being.

3.3.1 Setting Goals

SETTING GOALS IS AN essential part of self-management. By setting realistic and achievable goals, you can stay motivated and focused on improving your health. Start by identifying specific areas you want to work on, such as managing pain, improving mobility, or reducing stress. Break down your goals into smaller, manageable steps and create a plan to achieve them. Regularly review and adjust your goals as needed to ensure continued progress.

3.3.2 Developing a Self-Care Routine

DEVELOPING A SELF-CARE routine is vital for managing chronic conditions and promoting overall wellness. A self-care routine involves incorporating activities and practices into your daily life that support your physical, mental, and emotional well-being. This may include activities such as regular exercise, healthy eating, getting enough sleep, practicing relaxation techniques, and engaging in activities that bring you joy and fulfillment. By prioritizing self-care, you can better manage your condition and improve your overall quality of life.

3.3.3 Monitoring Symptoms

MONITORING YOUR SYMPTOMS is an essential part of self-management. By keeping track of your symptoms, you can identify patterns, triggers, and changes in your condition. This information can help you make informed decisions about your treatment plan and lifestyle choices. Use a symptom diary or a mobile app to record your symptoms, their severity, and any factors that may have contributed to them. Share this information with your healthcare provider during your appointments to facilitate effective communication and decision-making.

3.3.4 Medication Management

IF YOU ARE TAKING MEDICATIONS to manage your chronic condition, proper medication management is crucial. Follow your healthcare provider's instructions regarding medication dosage, timing, and any potential side effects. Set up a system to help you remember to take your medications, such as using pill organizers or setting reminders on your phone. Keep an updated list of all your medications, including over-the-counter drugs and supplements, and share it with your healthcare provider to avoid any potential drug interactions.

3.3.5 Stress Management

STRESS CAN HAVE A SIGNIFICANT impact on your overall well-being and can exacerbate the symptoms of chronic conditions. Developing effective stress management techniques can help you better cope with stress and improve your overall health. Explore different stress management techniques, such as deep breathing exercises, meditation, yoga, or engaging in hobbies and activities that help you relax. Find what works best for you, and incorporate these techniques into your daily routine.

3.3.6 Healthy Eating and Nutrition

PROPER NUTRITION PLAYS a vital role in managing chronic conditions and promoting overall wellness. Adopting a healthy eating plan can help you maintain a healthy weight, manage your condition, and reduce the risk of complications. Consult with a registered dietitian or healthcare provider to develop a personalized eating plan that meets your specific needs. Focus on consuming a balanced diet that includes a variety of fruits, vegetables, whole grains, lean proteins, and healthy fats. Limit the intake of processed foods, sugary beverages, and foods high in saturated and trans fats.

3.3.7 Regular Exercise

REGULAR EXERCISE IS beneficial for managing chronic conditions and improving overall health. Engaging in physical activity can help reduce symptoms, improve mobility, boost mood, and enhance overall well-being. Consult with your healthcare provider to determine the most suitable exercise program for your condition. Aim for a combination of aerobic exercises, strength training, and flexibility exercises. Start slowly and gradually increase the intensity and duration of your workouts. Listen to your body and modify your exercise routine as needed to avoid overexertion or injury.

3.3.8 Seeking Support

MANAGING A CHRONIC condition can be challenging, and seeking support is essential. Reach out to friends, family, or support groups who can provide emotional support and understanding. Consider joining online communities or support groups specific to your condition, where you can connect with others facing similar challenges. Additionally, don't hesitate to seek professional support from therapists, counselors, or healthcare providers who specialize in your condition. They can provide guidance, resources, and strategies to help you effectively manage your condition and improve your overall well-being.

3.3.9 Regular Check-ups and Communication with Healthcare Providers

REGULAR CHECK-UPS AND open communication with your healthcare providers are crucial for effective self-management. Schedule regular appointments with your primary care physician and any specialists involved in your care. Use these appointments to discuss any concerns, ask questions, and review your treatment plan. Be proactive in sharing any changes in your symptoms, medication side effects, or lifestyle modifications. Your healthcare providers can provide valuable guidance, adjust your treatment plan as needed, and ensure you are on the right track towards optimal health and well-being.

By implementing these self-management strategies, you can take an active role in managing your chronic condition and improving your overall wellness. Remember, self-management is a continuous process, and it may take time to find what works best for you. Stay committed, be patient with yourself, and celebrate your progress along the way. With dedication and perseverance, you can achieve a higher level of well-being and live a fulfilling life despite your chronic condition.

3.4 Support and Resources

When it comes to managing your health and well-being, having access to support and resources is essential. Whether you are dealing with a chronic condition or simply trying to maintain a healthy lifestyle, knowing where to turn for assistance can make all the difference. In this section, we will explore the various support systems and resources available to help you on your wellness journey.

3.4.1 Healthcare Professionals

ONE OF THE MOST IMPORTANT sources of support for managing your health is healthcare professionals. These individuals have the knowledge and expertise to provide you with the guidance and care you need. Depending on your specific needs, you may work with a primary care physician, a specialist, or a team of healthcare providers.

Your primary care physician is often your first point of contact for any health concerns. They can provide routine check-ups, preventive care, and general medical advice. If you have a chronic condition, you may also be referred to a specialist who has specialized knowledge and experience in managing your specific condition.

In addition to physicians, there are other healthcare professionals who can play a role in supporting your wellness. These may include nurses, nurse practitioners, dietitians, physical therapists, mental health professionals, and pharmacists. Each of these professionals brings a unique set of skills and expertise to help you manage your health effectively.

3.4.2 Support Groups

SUPPORT GROUPS CAN be a valuable resource for individuals dealing with chronic conditions or specific health challenges. These groups provide a safe and supportive environment where you can connect with others who are facing similar experiences. Sharing your journey with others who understand can provide emotional support, practical advice, and a sense of community.

Support groups can take many forms, including in-person meetings, online forums, and virtual communities. Some support groups are led by healthcare professionals, while others are peer-led. Regardless of the format, support groups offer a space for sharing experiences, learning from others, and finding encouragement and inspiration.

3.4.3 Online Resources

THE INTERNET HAS REVOLUTIONIZED the way we access information, and this includes health-related resources. Online resources can provide a wealth of information on a wide range of health topics, from general wellness tips to specific conditions and treatments. However, it is important to ensure that the information you find online is reliable and evidence-based.

When searching for health information online, look for reputable sources, such as government health websites, academic institutions, and professional organizations. These sources often provide accurate and up-to-date information that is backed by scientific research. It is also a good idea to consult with your healthcare provider to verify the information you find online and to get personalized advice.

In addition to informational websites, there are also online tools and apps that can help you track your health, set goals, and manage your wellness. These tools can range from fitness trackers and meal planning apps to symptom trackers and medication reminders. Exploring these resources can provide you with additional support and motivation on your wellness journey.

3.4.4 Community Programs and Services

MANY COMMUNITIES OFFER programs and services that are designed to support the health and well-being of their residents. These programs can vary widely, but they often include initiatives such as health screenings, wellness workshops, exercise classes, and support groups. These resources are typically provided by local government agencies, community organizations, and healthcare institutions.

Community programs and services can be a valuable source of support, particularly for individuals who may not have access to other resources. They often provide low-cost or free services and are designed to meet the specific needs of the community. These programs can not only help you improve your health but also connect you with others who share your goals and challenges.

3.4.5 Health Insurance and Financial Assistance

MANAGING YOUR HEALTH and accessing necessary care can sometimes be costly. Health insurance can help alleviate some of these financial burdens by covering a portion of your healthcare expenses. If you have health insurance, it is important to understand your coverage and benefits. Familiarize yourself with the terms of your policy, including any deductibles, copayments, and limitations.

If you do not have health insurance or if your insurance does not cover certain services, there may be financial assistance programs available to help. These programs can vary depending on your location and circumstances. Some options to explore include government assistance programs, charitable organizations, and patient assistance programs offered by pharmaceutical companies.

3.4.6 Family and Friends

NEVER UNDERESTIMATE the power of a strong support system. Family and friends can play a crucial role in supporting your wellness journey. They can provide emotional support, help with practical tasks, and serve as a sounding board for your concerns and challenges. Having someone to lean on can make a significant difference in your overall well-being.

Don't hesitate to reach out to your loved ones and let them know how they can support you. Whether it's accompanying you to medical appointments, helping with household chores, or simply lending a listening ear, their support can be invaluable. Remember, you don't have to face your health challenges alone.

Conclusion

Support and resources are essential for maintaining and improving your health and well-being. From healthcare professionals to support groups, online resources to community programs, there are numerous avenues to explore. Take advantage of these resources and empower yourself to live a healthier and happier life. Remember, you are not alone on your wellness journey.

Creating a Safe Environment

4.1 Home Safety

Your home should be a sanctuary, a place where you feel safe and secure. However, accidents can happen anywhere, even in the comfort of your own home. It is essential to take proactive measures to ensure the safety of yourself and your loved ones. This section will provide you with valuable information and practical tips on how to create a safe environment in your home.

4.1.1 General Safety Tips

- Keep your home well-lit. Adequate lighting is crucial for preventing accidents. Make sure all areas of your home are well-lit, especially stairways, hallways, and entrances. Install nightlights in bedrooms, bathrooms, and other areas that may be accessed during the night.

- Clear clutter: Remove any unnecessary items or clutter from walkways and stairs. Clutter can increase the risk of tripping and falling. Keep floors clear of toys, shoes, and other objects that may pose a hazard.

• Secure rugs and carpets: Use non-slip mats or double-sided tape to secure rugs and carpets to the floor. This will prevent them from slipping and causing falls.

• Install handrails: Install handrails on both sides of staircases to provide support and stability. Ensure that the handrails are securely attached and at a comfortable height.

• Use non-slip surfaces: Place non-slip mats or adhesive strips in the bathtub, shower, and on bathroom floors to prevent slips and falls. Additionally, consider using non-slip mats in the kitchen and other areas where water or spills may occur.

• Keep cords and wires out of the way: Secure cords and wires along walls or use cord covers to prevent tripping hazards. Avoid running cords under rugs or furniture.

• Install smoke detectors and carbon monoxide detectors. Place smoke detectors on every level of your home and near sleeping areas. Test them regularly and replace batteries as needed. Additionally, install carbon monoxide detectors near bedrooms and fuel-burning appliances.

• Keep emergency numbers accessible. Post emergency numbers, including poison control, fire

department, and ambulance, in a visible location.
Save these numbers on your phone as well.

4.1.2 Kitchen Safety

THE KITCHEN IS OFTEN the heart of the home, but it
can also be a place where accidents occur. Follow these tips to
ensure kitchen safety:

- Keep knives and sharp objects out of reach. Store
knives and other sharp objects in a secure drawer or
knife block. Keep them out of the reach of children.

- Use caution when handling hot objects. Use oven
mitts or pot holders when handling hot pots, pans,
or dishes. Avoid placing hot items on unstable
surfaces.

- Keep flammable objects away from the stove. Keep
flammable objects such as dish towels, paper towels,
and curtains away from the stove. This will reduce
the risk of fires.

- Use caution when using appliances. Follow the
manufacturer's instructions when using kitchen
appliances. Unplug appliances when they are not in
use.

- Practice safe food handling. Wash your hands
thoroughly before handling food. Store food at the
appropriate temperatures to prevent foodborne

illnesses. Clean cutting boards and utensils after each use.

4.1.3 Bathroom Safety

THE BATHROOM CAN BE a hazardous area due to wet surfaces and slippery floors. Take the following precautions to ensure bathroom safety:

- Install grab bars: Install grab bars near the toilet, bathtub, and shower to provide support and stability. Make sure they are securely attached to the wall.

- Use non-slip mats: Place non-slip mats or adhesive strips in the bathtub, shower, and on bathroom floors to prevent slips and falls.

- Adjust water temperature: Set your water heater to a safe temperature to prevent scalding. Test the water temperature before getting into the shower or bath.

- Store medications safely. Keep medications out of reach of children and store them in a secure cabinet. Dispose of expired or unused medications properly.

4.1.4 Bedroom Safety

YOUR BEDROOM SHOULD be a safe and comfortable space for rest and relaxation. Consider the following tips to ensure bedroom safety:

• Install smoke detectors: Place smoke detectors near sleeping areas and test them regularly.

• Use nightlights: Install nightlights in bedrooms, hallways, and bathrooms to prevent falls during the night.

• Keep a phone nearby: Keep a phone or mobile device within reach in case of emergencies.

• Ensure a comfortable sleeping environment. Use a mattress and pillows that provide adequate support. Keep the room at a comfortable temperature and ensure proper ventilation.

4.1.5 Childproofing

IF YOU HAVE YOUNG CHILDREN in your home, it is essential to take additional measures to ensure their safety. Consider the following childproofing tips:

• Install safety gates: Use safety gates at the top and bottom of staircases to prevent falls.

• Secure furniture: Anchor heavy furniture, such as bookshelves and dressers, to the wall to prevent tipping.

• Keep small objects out of reach: Keep small objects, such as coins, batteries, and small toys, out of reach of young children to prevent choking hazards.

• Cover electrical outlets: Use outlet covers or safety plugs to prevent children from inserting objects into electrical outlets.

• Lock cabinets and drawers: Install childproof locks on cabinets and drawers that contain hazardous substances or sharp objects.

By implementing these home safety measures, you can create a secure environment for yourself and your loved ones. Remember to regularly review and update your safety practices to ensure ongoing protection.

4.2 Workplace Safety

Workplace safety is a crucial aspect of overall wellness and care. Many individuals spend a significant portion of their lives in the workplace, making it essential to prioritize safety in this environment. By creating a safe and healthy workplace, employers can protect their employees from potential hazards and promote their well-being. In this section, we will explore the importance of workplace safety, common workplace hazards, and strategies for creating a safe work environment.

4.2.1 The Importance of Workplace Safety

WORKPLACE SAFETY IS not only important for the well-being of employees but also for the success of the organization. When employees feel safe and secure in their work environment, they are more likely to be productive, engaged, and satisfied with their jobs. On the other hand, a lack of workplace safety can lead to accidents, injuries, and even fatalities, resulting in physical, emotional, and financial consequences for both employees and employers.

Employers have a legal and moral responsibility to provide a safe work environment for their employees. This includes identifying and addressing potential hazards, implementing safety protocols and procedures, and providing appropriate training and resources. By prioritizing workplace safety, employers can reduce the risk of accidents and injuries, minimize absenteeism and turnover, and enhance the overall well-being of their workforce.

4.2.2 Common Workplace Hazards

WORKPLACES CAN PRESENT a variety of hazards that can compromise the safety and well-being of employees. It is essential for employers to be aware of these hazards and take appropriate measures to mitigate them. Some common workplace hazards include:

1. Physical Hazards: These hazards include slips, trips, and falls; ergonomic issues; noise exposure; and exposure to extreme temperatures. Employers should ensure that the workplace is properly maintained, provide ergonomic equipment and training, implement measures to reduce noise levels, and establish protocols for working in extreme temperatures.

2. Chemical Hazards: Chemical hazards can arise from exposure to toxic substances, such as cleaning agents, solvents, and pesticides. Employers should provide employees with appropriate personal protective equipment (PPE), ensure proper storage and handling of chemicals, and provide training on the safe use of hazardous substances.

3. Biological Hazards: Biological hazards can include exposure to infectious diseases, such as viruses and

bacteria. Employers should implement measures to prevent the spread of diseases, such as regular cleaning and disinfection, providing access to hand hygiene facilities, and promoting vaccination programs.

4. Psychological Hazards: Psychological hazards can arise from workplace stress, bullying, harassment, and violence. Employers should promote a positive work culture, provide resources for stress management, implement anti-bullying and harassment policies, and establish protocols for addressing workplace violence.

4.2.3 Strategies for Creating a Safe Work Environment

CREATING A SAFE WORK environment requires a proactive approach that involves the participation and collaboration of both employers and employees. Here are some strategies for promoting workplace safety:

1. Risk Assessment: Conduct regular risk assessments to identify potential hazards in the workplace. This can involve inspecting the physical environment, reviewing work processes, and consulting with employees. By understanding the risks, employers can implement appropriate control measures to minimize or eliminate them.

2. Training and Education: Provide comprehensive training and education programs for employees on workplace safety. This should include information on hazard identification, proper use of equipment and machinery, emergency procedures, and the

importance of reporting incidents and near misses. Regular refresher training should also be conducted to reinforce safety practices.

3. Safety Policies and Procedures: Develop and implement clear safety policies and procedures that outline expectations and responsibilities for both employers and employees. These policies should cover areas such as personal protective equipment, emergency response, incident reporting, and hazard control measures. Regularly review and update these policies to ensure their effectiveness.

4. Safety Equipment and Facilities: Provide employees with the necessary safety equipment and facilities to perform their jobs safely. This may include personal protective equipment (PPE), such as gloves, goggles, and helmets, as well as safety signage, fire extinguishers, first aid kits, and emergency exits. Regularly inspect and maintain this equipment and facility to ensure their functionality.

5. Employee Engagement: Encourage employee involvement and engagement in workplace safety initiatives. This can be achieved through safety committees, regular safety meetings, and open communication channels. Employees should be encouraged to report hazards, near misses, and incidents, and their feedback should be valued and acted upon.

6. Continuous Improvement: Regularly evaluate and review workplace safety practices to identify areas for improvement. This can involve analyzing incident

reports, conducting safety audits, and seeking feedback from employees. By continuously striving for improvement, employers can create a culture of safety and ensure the well-being of their workforce.

Remember, workplace safety is a shared responsibility that requires the commitment and cooperation of both employers and employees. By implementing these strategies and fostering a culture of safety, organizations can create a work environment that promotes wellness, care, and productivity.

4.3 Community Safety

Community safety plays a crucial role in promoting overall wellness and ensuring the well-being of individuals and families. A safe community provides a supportive environment where people can thrive and lead healthy lives. In this section, we will explore various aspects of community safety and discuss strategies to enhance safety in your neighborhood.

4.3.1 Neighborhood Watch Programs

NEIGHBORHOOD WATCH programs are an effective way to promote community safety and prevent crime. These programs involve residents working together to keep an eye out for suspicious activities and report them to the appropriate authorities. By actively participating in a neighborhood watch program, you can contribute to creating a safer environment for everyone.

To start a neighborhood watch program in your community, follow these steps:

1. **Gather interested residents:** Reach out to your neighbors and gauge their interest in starting a neighborhood watch program. Encourage them to attend an initial meeting to discuss the program's goals and objectives.

2. **Contact local law enforcement:** Get in touch with your local

police department or community policing officer to seek their guidance and support. They can provide valuable resources, training, and advice on setting up an effective neighborhood watch program.

3. **Establish communication channels:** Create a system for sharing information and communicating with other members of the neighborhood watch program. This can include setting up a dedicated email group, a social media page, or using a neighborhood watch app.

4. **Organize regular meetings:** Schedule regular meetings to discuss safety concerns, share updates, and plan community events. These meetings provide an opportunity for residents to connect, exchange ideas, and collaborate on initiatives to improve community safety.

5. **Educate and train:** Arrange educational sessions and training workshops for members of the neighborhood watch program. These sessions can cover topics such as crime prevention, emergency preparedness, and personal safety.

6. **Engage with the community:** Foster a sense of community by organizing events and activities that bring residents together. This can include neighborhood clean-up days, block parties, or community awareness campaigns.

By actively participating in a neighborhood watch program, you can contribute to creating a safer and more secure community for everyone.

4.3.2 Safe Public Spaces

PUBLIC SPACES ARE AN integral part of any community, providing opportunities for recreation, socialization, and relaxation. Ensuring the safety of these spaces is essential for promoting community wellness. Here are some strategies to enhance safety in public areas:

1. **Well-lit areas:** Adequate lighting is crucial in preventing crime and creating a sense of security. Encourage local authorities to install and maintain proper lighting in parks, playgrounds, and other public spaces.

2. **Regular maintenance:** Regular maintenance of public spaces is essential to prevent accidents and ensure a safe environment. Report any damaged equipment, broken sidewalks, or other hazards to the appropriate authorities.

3. **Security measures:** Install security cameras and alarms in high-risk areas to deter criminal activities. Work with local law enforcement to identify areas that require additional security measures and implement them accordingly.

4. **Community involvement:** Encourage community members to actively participate in the maintenance and upkeep of public spaces. Organize volunteer groups to clean up parks, plant trees, and create a sense of ownership and pride in these areas.

5. **Awareness campaigns:** Conduct awareness campaigns to educate the community about safety measures and encourage responsible behavior in public spaces. This can include distributing brochures, organizing workshops, or hosting community events focused on safety.

By implementing these strategies, you can help create safe and inviting public spaces that promote community well-being and encourage active participation.

4.3.3 Emergency Preparedness

BEING PREPARED FOR emergencies is crucial to ensuring the safety and well-being of individuals and communities. By taking proactive steps to prepare for emergencies, you can minimize the impact of disasters and protect yourself and your loved ones. Here are some key aspects of emergency preparedness:

1. **Create an emergency plan.** Develop a comprehensive emergency plan for your household. This plan should include evacuation routes, designated meeting points, and a communication strategy. Ensure that all family members are aware of the plan and practice it regularly.

2. **Assemble an emergency kit:** Put together an emergency kit that includes essential supplies such as food, water, medications, first aid supplies, flashlights, and batteries. Keep the kit in a readily accessible location, and regularly check and replenish its contents.

3. **Stay informed:** Stay informed about potential hazards and emergency situations in your area. Sign up for local emergency alerts and familiarize yourself with the emergency response procedures in your community.

4. **Community emergency response teams:** Consider joining or forming a community emergency response team (CERT). CERT members receive training in basic disaster response skills and can provide assistance to their neighbors during emergencies.

5. **Collaborate with neighbors:** Establish a network of neighbors who can support each other during emergencies. Share contact information, discuss emergency plans, and offer assistance to

those who may need it.

6. **Practice resilience:** Building resilience is essential to coping with and recovering from emergencies. Foster a sense of community and support by checking on your neighbors, offering assistance, and promoting a culture of preparedness.

By taking these steps, you can contribute to a safer and more resilient community where individuals are prepared to face emergencies and support one another in times of crisis.

Conclusion

C ommunity safety is a collective responsibility that requires the active participation and collaboration of individuals, families, and local authorities. By implementing strategies to enhance community safety, we can create an environment that promotes wellness, fosters a sense of belonging, and ensures the well-being of all community members. Remember, small actions can make a big difference in creating a safe and healthy community for everyone.

4.4 Emergency Preparedness

In times of crisis or unexpected events, being prepared can make all the difference. Emergency preparedness is an essential aspect of creating a safe environment for yourself and your loved ones. It involves taking proactive steps to minimize the impact of emergencies and ensure the well-being of everyone involved. This chapter will guide you through the necessary measures to prepare for emergencies effectively.

4.4.1 Understanding Emergency Preparedness

EMERGENCY PREPAREDNESS refers to the actions taken to anticipate, respond to, and recover from emergencies or disasters. These can include natural disasters such as hurricanes, earthquakes, and floods, or man-made emergencies like fires, chemical spills, or terrorist attacks. By understanding the potential risks and hazards in your area, you can better prepare for emergencies and protect yourself and your loved ones.

4.4.2 Assessing Risks and Hazards

THE FIRST STEP IN EMERGENCY preparedness is to assess the risks and hazards specific to your location. Research the common emergencies that occur in your area and understand their potential impact. This could include studying historical data, consulting local authorities, or using online resources. By identifying the potential risks, you can develop a plan that addresses these specific challenges.

4.4.3 Creating an Emergency Plan

DEVELOPING AN EMERGENCY plan is crucial to ensuring everyone's safety during a crisis. Start by discussing and involving all members of your household in the planning process. Consider the specific needs of children, elderly family members, or individuals with disabilities. Your emergency plan should include:

1. Communication: Establish a communication plan to stay connected with your family members during an emergency. Designate a meeting point and determine how you will communicate if traditional methods are unavailable. Consider using text messages, social media, or designated apps for emergency communication.

2. Evacuation Routes: Identify the safest evacuation routes in your area and establish alternative routes in case the primary ones are inaccessible. Familiarize yourself with local evacuation procedures and shelters. Ensure that everyone in your household knows the evacuation plan and where to meet if separated.

3. Emergency Contacts: Compile a list of emergency contacts, including local authorities, hospitals, and family members or friends who can provide assistance. Keep this list in a readily accessible location, and

ensure that everyone in your household knows where to find it.

4. Essential Supplies: Prepare an emergency supply kit that includes essential items such as non-perishable food, water, medications, first aid supplies, flashlights, batteries, and a battery-powered radio. Regularly check and update your emergency kit to ensure that all items are in working order and have not expired.

5. Important Documents: Make copies of important documents such as identification cards, passports, insurance policies, and medical records. Store these copies in a waterproof and fireproof container or keep them in a secure digital format. This will help facilitate the recovery process after an emergency.

6. Pet Preparedness: If you have pets, include them in your emergency plan. Ensure that you have enough food, water, medications, and supplies for your pets. Identify pet-friendly shelters or accommodations in case you need to evacuate.

4.4.4 Emergency Response and Recovery

DURING AN EMERGENCY, it is essential to remain calm and follow your emergency plan. Stay informed by listening to local authorities and emergency broadcasts for updates and instructions. If evacuation is necessary, leave immediately and follow the designated routes. Remember to take your emergency supply kit and important documents with you.

After the emergency has passed, focus on the recovery process. Assess the damage to your property and prioritize repairs or cleanup tasks. Contact your insurance company to report any damages and initiate the claims process if necessary. Seek assistance from local resources and support organizations if needed.

4.4.5 Community Involvement

EMERGENCY PREPAREDNESS is not just an individual responsibility; it is also a community effort. Get involved in your community's emergency preparedness initiatives, such as neighborhood watch programs or local emergency response teams. By working together, you can enhance the overall safety and resilience of your community.

4.4.6 Regular Review and Practice

EMERGENCY PREPAREDNESS plans should be regularly reviewed and practiced to ensure their effectiveness. Schedule regular drills with your household to practice evacuation procedures and communication methods. Update your emergency supply kit as needed, and replace any expired items. Stay informed about changes in local emergency procedures and adapt your plan accordingly.

By taking the time to prepare for emergencies, you can significantly reduce the impact they have on your life and the lives of those around you. Remember, being proactive and informed is the key to effectively managing emergencies and ensuring the safety and well-being of yourself and your loved ones.

Nutrition and Exercise

5.1 Importance of Nutrition

Nutrition plays a vital role in our overall health and well-being. It is the foundation of a healthy lifestyle and is essential for the proper functioning of our bodies. Good nutrition provides us with the necessary nutrients, vitamins, and minerals that our bodies need to function optimally. It helps to support our immune system, maintain a healthy weight, and reduce the risk of chronic diseases.

5.1.1 The Role of Nutrients

NUTRIENTS ARE SUBSTANCES found in food that are essential for our bodies to function properly. They can be divided into macronutrients and micronutrients. Macronutrients include carbohydrates, proteins, and fats, which provide us with energy. Micronutrients include vitamins and minerals, which are necessary for various bodily functions.

Carbohydrates are the body's main source of energy. They are found in foods such as grains, fruits, and vegetables. Proteins are essential for the growth, repair, and maintenance of body tissues. They are found in foods such as meat, fish, dairy products, and legumes. Fats are important for energy storage, insulation, and the absorption of fat-soluble vitamins. They are found in foods such as oils, nuts, and seeds.

Vitamins and minerals are essential for the proper functioning of our bodies. They help to support our immune system, regulate our metabolism, and maintain healthy bones, teeth, and skin. Vitamins are found in a variety of foods, including fruits, vegetables, and whole grains. Minerals are found in foods such as meat, dairy products, and leafy green vegetables.

5.1.2 The Benefits of a Balanced Diet

A BALANCED DIET IS one that provides all the necessary nutrients in the right proportions. It is important to consume a variety of foods from different food groups to ensure that we are getting all the nutrients our bodies need. A balanced diet has numerous benefits for our health and well-being.

One of the key benefits of a balanced diet is maintaining a healthy weight. When we consume a balanced diet, we are more likely to consume the right amount of calories for our bodies. This helps to prevent weight gain and reduce the risk of obesity, which is a major risk factor for many chronic diseases, including heart disease, diabetes, and certain types of cancer.

A balanced diet also helps to support our immune system. The nutrients in our food play a crucial role in supporting the immune system's ability to fight off infections and diseases. A diet rich in fruits, vegetables, whole grains, and lean proteins provides us with the necessary vitamins, minerals, and antioxidants that help to strengthen our immune system.

In addition, a balanced diet can help reduce the risk of chronic diseases. Many chronic diseases, such as heart disease, diabetes, and certain types of cancer, are linked to poor nutrition. Consuming a diet that is rich in fruits, vegetables, whole grains, and lean proteins can help reduce the risk of these diseases and promote overall health and well-being.

5.1.3 Making Healthy Food Choices

MAKING HEALTHY FOOD choices is an important part of maintaining a balanced diet. Here are some tips to help you make healthier choices:

1. Eat a variety of foods: Include a variety of fruits, vegetables, whole grains, lean proteins, and healthy fats in your diet. This will ensure that you are getting a wide range of nutrients.

2. Limit processed foods. Processed foods are often high in added sugars, unhealthy fats, and sodium. Try to limit your intake of processed foods and opt for whole, unprocessed foods whenever possible.

3. Watch your portion sizes: Pay attention to portion sizes and try to eat smaller, more frequent meals throughout the day. This can help to prevent overeating and promote better digestion.

4. Stay hydrated: Drink plenty of water throughout the day to stay hydrated. Water is essential for many bodily functions and can help to curb hunger and prevent overeating.

5. Limit sugary drinks: Sugary drinks, such as soda and fruit juices, are high in added sugars and can contribute to weight gain and other health issues. Opt for water, herbal tea, or unsweetened beverages instead.

6. Cook at home: Cooking at home allows you to have

more control over the ingredients in your meals. Try to cook meals from scratch using fresh, whole ingredients whenever possible.

7. Practice mindful eating: Pay attention to your body's hunger and fullness cues. Eat slowly and savor each bite, and stop eating when you feel satisfied, not overly full.

By making these small changes to your eating habits, you can improve your nutrition and overall health.

5.1.4 The Role of Nutrition in Disease Prevention

PROPER NUTRITION PLAYS a crucial role in preventing various diseases and promoting overall health. A healthy diet can help reduce the risk of chronic diseases such as heart disease, diabetes, and certain types of cancer.

Heart disease is the leading cause of death worldwide, and poor nutrition is a major risk factor. A diet high in saturated and trans fats, cholesterol, and sodium can contribute to high blood pressure, high cholesterol levels, and obesity, all of which are risk factors for heart disease. On the other hand, a diet rich in fruits, vegetables, whole grains, lean proteins, and healthy fats can help reduce the risk of heart disease.

Diabetes is a chronic condition characterized by high blood sugar levels. Poor nutrition and unhealthy eating habits can contribute to the development of type 2 diabetes. Consuming a diet that is high in refined carbohydrates, added sugars, and unhealthy fats can lead to weight gain and insulin resistance, both of which are risk factors for diabetes. A balanced diet that is rich in whole grains, fruits, vegetables, lean proteins, and healthy fats can help to prevent and manage diabetes.

Certain types of cancer, such as colorectal, breast, and prostate cancer, have been linked to poor nutrition. A diet that is high in processed meats, saturated fats, and added sugars can increase the risk of these types of cancer. On the other hand, a diet that is rich in fruits, vegetables, whole grains, and lean proteins can help reduce the risk of cancer.

In conclusion, nutrition plays a crucial role in our overall health and well-being. A balanced diet that is rich in fruits, vegetables, whole grains, lean proteins, and healthy fats can help to prevent illness, maintain a healthy weight, and reduce the risk of chronic diseases. By making healthy food choices and practicing mindful eating, we can improve our nutrition and live a healthier, happier life.

5.2 Healthy Eating Guidelines

Maintaining a healthy diet is essential for overall wellness and plays a crucial role in preventing chronic diseases, promoting proper growth and development, and supporting optimal physical and mental functioning. In this section, we will explore the key principles and guidelines for healthy eating that can help you make informed choices about your diet and improve your overall well-being.

5.2.1 Balancing Macronutrients

A BALANCED DIET CONSISTS of the right proportions of macronutrients, which include carbohydrates, proteins, and fats. These macronutrients provide the body with energy and are essential for various bodily functions.

Carbohydrates are the body's primary source of energy and should make up the majority of your daily calorie intake. Choose complex carbohydrates such as whole grains, fruits, and vegetables, as they provide essential nutrients and fiber.

Proteins are essential for building and repairing tissues, supporting immune function, and producing enzymes and hormones. Include a variety of lean protein sources, such as poultry, fish, beans, legumes, and nuts, in your diet.

Fats are important for hormone production, insulation, and the absorption of fat-soluble vitamins. Opt for healthy fats like avocados, nuts, seeds, and olive oil while limiting saturated and trans fats found in fried foods, processed snacks, and fatty meats.

5.2.2 Portion Control

MAINTAINING PROPER portion sizes is crucial for managing weight and preventing overeating. It's important to be mindful of the quantity of food you consume to ensure you're meeting your nutritional needs without exceeding your energy requirements.

Use visual cues to estimate portion sizes. For example, a serving of meat should be about the size of a deck of cards, a serving of grains or starchy vegetables should be about the size of your fist, and a serving of cheese should be about the size of your thumb.

Avoid eating directly from large packages or containers, as it can lead to mindless eating. Instead, portion out your food onto a plate or bowl to help you better gauge how much you're consuming.

Listen to your body's hunger and fullness cues. Eat slowly and stop eating when you feel comfortably satisfied, rather than waiting until you're overly full.

5.2.3 Variety and Moderation

EATING A VARIETY OF foods ensures that you receive a wide range of essential nutrients. Aim to include foods from all food groups in your diet, including fruits, vegetables, whole grains, lean proteins, and healthy fats.

Moderation is key when it comes to indulging in less nutritious foods. While it's important to enjoy your favorite treats occasionally, it's best to limit foods that are high in added sugars, sodium, and unhealthy fats. Opt for healthier alternatives whenever possible.

5.2.4 Hydration

STAYING HYDRATED IS essential for overall health and well-being. Water is the best choice for hydration, but other beverages such as herbal tea, unsweetened coffee, and low-fat milk can also contribute to your daily fluid intake.

Aim to drink at least 8 cups (64 ounces) of water per day, or more if you're physically active or in a hot climate. Remember to listen to your body's thirst signals and drink water throughout the day to stay adequately hydrated.

5.2.5 Mindful Eating

PRACTICING MINDFUL eating can help you develop a healthier relationship with food and improve your overall eating habits. Mindful eating involves paying attention to the present moment, savoring each bite, and being aware of your body's hunger and fullness cues.

Avoid distractions while eating, such as watching TV or using electronic devices. Instead, focus on the taste, texture, and aroma of your food.

Eat slowly, and chew your food thoroughly. This allows your body to properly digest and absorb nutrients while giving your brain time to register feelings of fullness.

Listen to your body's hunger and fullness cues. Eat when you're hungry and stop when you're satisfied, rather than eating out of boredom or emotional reasons.

5.2.6 Meal Planning and Preparation

MEAL PLANNING AND PREPARATION can help you make healthier food choices and save time and money. By planning your meals in advance, you can ensure that you have nutritious options readily available and avoid relying on unhealthy convenience foods.

Start by creating a weekly meal plan that includes a variety of foods from different food groups. Consider your schedule, dietary preferences, and nutritional needs when planning your meals.

Make a shopping list based on your meal plan and stick to it when grocery shopping. This can help you avoid impulse purchases and ensure that you have all the ingredients you need for your planned meals.

Set aside time each week for meal preparation. This may involve chopping vegetables, cooking grains, or prepping ingredients for future meals. Having pre-prepared components can make it easier to assemble healthy meals throughout the week.

5.2.7 Seeking Professional Guidance

IF YOU HAVE SPECIFIC dietary needs or health concerns, it may be beneficial to seek guidance from a registered dietitian or nutritionist. These professionals can provide personalized recommendations and help you develop a nutrition plan that meets your unique needs and goals.

A registered dietitian can help you navigate food allergies or intolerances, manage chronic conditions, optimize sports performance, or achieve weight loss or weight gain goals. They can also provide guidance on specific dietary patterns, such as vegetarian or vegan diets.

Remember that everyone's nutritional needs are different, and what works for one person may not work for another. It's important to listen to your body, make informed choices, and seek professional guidance when needed.

By following these healthy eating guidelines, you can nourish your body with the nutrients it needs to thrive. Remember that small changes over time can lead to significant improvements in your overall health and well-being. Start incorporating these principles into your daily life and enjoy the benefits of a balanced and nutritious diet.

5.3 Physical Activity and Exercise

Physical activity and exercise play a crucial role in maintaining overall health and well-being. Engaging in regular physical activity not only helps to improve physical fitness but also has numerous benefits for mental and emotional well-being. In this section, we will explore the importance of physical activity and exercise, different types of exercises, and how to incorporate them into your daily routine.

5.3.1 Benefits of Physical Activity

REGULAR PHYSICAL ACTIVITY offers a wide range of benefits for both the body and mind. Here are some of the key benefits:

1. **Improved cardiovascular health**: Engaging in aerobic exercises such as walking, running, swimming, or cycling helps to strengthen the heart and improve blood circulation, reducing the risk of heart disease.

2. **Weight management**: Physical activity helps to burn calories and maintain a healthy weight. Combined with a balanced diet, regular exercise can assist in weight loss and prevent obesity.

3. **Increased muscle strength and flexibility**: Strength training exercises, such as weightlifting or resistance training, help to build and tone muscles, improving overall strength and

flexibility.

4. **Enhanced mental well-being**: Physical activity stimulates the release of endorphins, also known as "feel-good" hormones, which can help reduce stress, anxiety, and symptoms of depression. Regular exercise can also improve sleep quality and boost self-esteem.

5. **Reduced risk of chronic diseases**: Regular physical activity has been shown to lower the risk of developing chronic conditions such as type 2 diabetes, certain types of cancer, and osteoporosis.

6. **Improved cognitive function**: Exercise has been linked to improved cognitive function, including better memory, attention, and problem-solving skills. It can also reduce the risk of age-related cognitive decline and improve overall brain health.

5.3.2 Types of Physical Activity

THERE ARE FOUR MAIN types of physical activity that should be incorporated into a well-rounded exercise routine:

1. **Aerobic exercise**: This type of exercise involves continuous, rhythmic movements that increase the heart rate and breathing. Examples include brisk walking, jogging, swimming, dancing, and cycling. Aim for at least 150 minutes of moderate-intensity aerobic activity or 75 minutes of vigorous-intensity aerobic activity per week.

2. **Strength training**: Strength training exercises focus on building and toning muscles. This can be done using free weights, weight machines, resistance bands, or bodyweight exercises such as push-ups, squats, and lunges. Aim for two or more days of strength training exercises per week, targeting all major muscle groups.

3. **Flexibility exercises**: Flexibility exercises help to improve joint mobility and prevent injuries. Examples include stretching exercises, yoga, and Pilates. Incorporate flexibility exercises into your routine at least two to three times per week.

4. **Balance exercises**: Balance exercises are important, especially for older adults, as they help to improve stability and reduce the risk of falls. Examples include standing on one leg, heel-to-toe walking, and Tai Chi. Aim for balance exercises at least three times per week.

5.3.3 Incorporating Physical Activity into Your Routine

FINDING WAYS TO INCORPORATE physical activity into your daily routine can help make it a sustainable and enjoyable habit. Here are some tips to help you get started:

1. **Set realistic goals**: Start with small, achievable goals and gradually increase the duration and intensity of your workouts. This will help you stay motivated and avoid burnout or injuries.

2. **Find activities you enjoy**: Choose activities that you genuinely enjoy, whether it's dancing, hiking, swimming, or playing a sport. This will make it easier to stick to your exercise routine and make it more enjoyable.

3. **Make it a priority.** Schedule your workouts like any other important appointment and treat them as non-negotiable. Set aside dedicated time for physical activity and make it a priority in your daily routine.

4. **Mix it up**: Vary your workouts to keep things interesting and prevent boredom. Try different types of exercises, join group classes, or explore outdoor activities to add variety to your

routine.

5. **Stay consistent**: Aim for at least 150 minutes of moderate-intensity aerobic activity or 75 minutes of vigorous-intensity aerobic activity per week, along with strength training exercises and flexibility exercises. Consistency is key to reaping the benefits of physical activity.

6. **Listen to your body**: Pay attention to how your body feels during and after exercise. If you experience pain or discomfort, modify or stop the activity, and consult a healthcare professional if necessary.

7. **Stay hydrated**: Drink plenty of water before, during, and after exercise to stay hydrated and maintain optimal performance.

Remember, it's important to consult with your healthcare provider before starting any new exercise program, especially if you have any underlying health conditions or concerns.

Incorporating regular physical activity and exercise into your daily routine is a powerful way to improve your overall health and well-being. By making it a priority and finding activities you enjoy, you can create a sustainable and fulfilling exercise routine that will benefit you for years to come. So, lace up your sneakers, grab a water bottle, and get moving towards a healthier and happier you!

5.4 Maintaining a Healthy Weight

Maintaining a healthy weight is an essential aspect of overall wellness. It not only helps to prevent various health conditions but also improves your quality of life. Achieving and maintaining a healthy weight requires a combination of healthy eating habits, regular physical activity, and a positive mindset. In this section, we will explore the importance of maintaining a healthy weight, the factors that contribute to weight gain, and practical tips for achieving and sustaining a healthy weight.

5.4.1 Understanding the Importance of Maintaining a Healthy Weight

MAINTAINING A HEALTHY weight is crucial for your overall well-being. Excess weight can increase the risk of various health problems, including heart disease, diabetes, high blood pressure, and certain types of cancer. It can also lead to joint pain, sleep apnea, and reduced mobility. On the other hand, maintaining a healthy weight can improve your energy levels, enhance your mood, boost your self-confidence, and increase your longevity.

5.4.2 Factors Contributing to Weight Gain

WEIGHT GAIN CAN BE influenced by a variety of factors, including genetics, lifestyle choices, and environmental factors. Understanding these factors can help you make informed decisions and take proactive steps towards maintaining a healthy weight.

Genetics

GENETICS PLAYS A ROLE in determining your body type and metabolism. Some individuals may have a genetic predisposition to gain weight more easily than others. However, genetics alone do not determine your weight. By adopting healthy lifestyle habits, you can still achieve and maintain a healthy weight, regardless of your genetic makeup.

Lifestyle Choices

UNHEALTHY LIFESTYLE choices, such as a sedentary lifestyle, poor dietary habits, and excessive consumption of processed foods and sugary beverages, can contribute to weight gain. Lack of physical activity and excessive calorie intake can lead to an energy imbalance where the calories consumed exceed the calories burned, resulting in weight gain.

Emotional Factors

EMOTIONAL FACTORS, such as stress, boredom, and emotional eating, can also contribute to weight gain. Many individuals turn to food as a way to cope with their emotions, leading to overeating and weight gain. It is important to develop healthy coping mechanisms and find alternative ways to manage stress and emotions.

Environmental Factors

THE ENVIRONMENT IN which you live can also influence your weight. Factors such as easy access to unhealthy food options, sedentary work environments, and a lack of safe spaces for physical activity can contribute to weight gain. Creating a supportive environment that promotes healthy eating and regular physical activity is essential for maintaining a healthy weight.

5.4.3 Tips for Achieving and Sustaining a Healthy Weight

ACHIEVING AND SUSTAINING a healthy weight requires a holistic approach that encompasses both dietary and lifestyle changes. Here are some practical tips to help you maintain a healthy weight:

1. Eat a balanced diet.

FOCUS ON CONSUMING a variety of nutrient-dense foods, including fruits, vegetables, whole grains, lean proteins, and healthy fats. Avoid or limit the intake of processed foods, sugary snacks, and beverages high in added sugars. Practice portion control and mindful eating to avoid overeating.

2. Stay hydrated.

DRINK AN ADEQUATE AMOUNT of water throughout the day to stay hydrated. Water can help curb your appetite, boost your metabolism, and aid in digestion. Avoid sugary drinks and opt for water, herbal tea, or infused water instead.

3. Engage in regular physical activity.

INCORPORATE REGULAR physical activity into your daily routine. Aim for at least 150 minutes of moderate-intensity aerobic activity or 75 minutes of vigorous-intensity aerobic activity per week. Additionally, include strength-training exercises to build muscle and increase your metabolism.

4. Practice Portion Control

BE MINDFUL OF PORTION sizes and avoid oversized servings. Use smaller plates and bowls to help control portion sizes. Listen to your body's hunger and fullness cues and stop eating when you feel satisfied, not overly full.

5. Get adequate sleep.

PRIORITIZE GETTING enough sleep each night. Lack of sleep can disrupt your hormones, leading to increased appetite and cravings for unhealthy foods. Aim for 7-9 hours of quality sleep per night.

6. Manage stress

FIND HEALTHY WAYS TO manage stress, such as by practicing relaxation techniques, engaging in hobbies, or seeking support from friends and family. Stress can lead to emotional eating and weight gain, so it is important to develop effective stress management strategies.

7. Seek support.

CONSIDER SEEKING SUPPORT from a healthcare professional or a registered dietitian who can provide personalized guidance and support on your weight management journey. They can help you set realistic goals, develop a tailored meal plan, and provide ongoing support and accountability.

8. Stay consistent.

REMEMBER THAT MAINTAINING a healthy weight is a lifelong commitment. Stay consistent with your healthy eating habits and physical activity routine. Celebrate your progress and focus on the positive changes you are making for your overall well-being.

By implementing these tips and making sustainable lifestyle changes, you can achieve and maintain a healthy weight. Remember, it's not just about the number on the scale but about nourishing your body, improving your health, and enhancing your overall quality of life.

Mental and Emotional Well-being

6.1 Understanding Mental Health

Mental health is an essential aspect of overall well-being. It encompasses our emotional, psychological, and social well-being, affecting how we think, feel, and act. Just like physical health, mental health is crucial for leading a fulfilling and productive life. Understanding mental health is the first step towards promoting and maintaining optimal well-being.

6.1.1 The Importance of Mental Health

MENTAL HEALTH PLAYS a vital role in our daily lives. It affects how we handle stress, make decisions, and interact with others. Good mental health allows us to cope with the challenges and pressures of life, maintain healthy relationships, and achieve our goals. On the other hand, poor mental health can lead to various difficulties, including decreased productivity, strained relationships, and even physical health problems.

6.1.2 Common Mental Health Conditions

THERE ARE SEVERAL COMMON mental health conditions that individuals may experience at some point in their lives. These conditions can range from mild to severe and can have a significant impact on a person's well-being. Some of the most prevalent mental health conditions include:

1. Anxiety Disorders: Anxiety disorders involve excessive worry, fear, or unease that can interfere with daily life. Generalized anxiety disorder, panic disorder, and social anxiety disorder are examples of anxiety disorders.

2. Depression: Depression is a mood disorder characterized by persistent feelings of sadness, a loss of interest, and a lack of motivation. It can affect a person's ability to function well and enjoy life.

3. Bipolar Disorder: Bipolar disorder is a condition marked by extreme mood swings, ranging from periods of intense euphoria (mania) to episodes of deep depression.

4. Schizophrenia: Schizophrenia is a chronic mental disorder that affects a person's perception of reality, thoughts, emotions, and behavior. It often involves hallucinations, delusions, and disorganized thinking.

5. Eating Disorders: Eating disorders, such as anorexia nervosa, bulimia nervosa, and binge-eating disorder, involve unhealthy eating behaviors and a distorted body image.

6. Substance Use Disorders: Substance use disorders occur when the use of drugs or alcohol leads to significant impairment in daily functioning and causes distress.

6.1.3 Factors Influencing Mental Health

SEVERAL FACTORS CAN influence an individual's mental health. These factors can be biological, psychological, or environmental in nature. Understanding these influences can help individuals take proactive steps to promote their mental well-being. Some common factors that can impact mental health include:

1. Biological Factors: Genetic predisposition, brain chemistry, and hormonal imbalances can contribute to the development of mental health conditions.
2. Psychological Factors: Past experiences, trauma, and coping mechanisms can influence mental health. Additionally, personality traits and individual resilience play a role in how individuals respond to stress and adversity.
3. Environmental Factors: Social and cultural factors, such as family dynamics, socioeconomic status, and access to support systems, can impact mental health. Additionally, exposure to violence, discrimination, or ongoing stressors can contribute to mental health challenges.

6.1.4 Promoting Mental Health

PROMOTING MENTAL HEALTH involves taking proactive steps to maintain and enhance well-being. Here are some strategies that can help individuals promote their mental health:

1. Self-Care: Engaging in self-care activities, such as

practicing relaxation techniques, getting enough sleep, and engaging in hobbies, can help reduce stress and improve overall well-being.

2. Healthy Lifestyle: Adopting a healthy lifestyle that includes regular physical activity, a balanced diet, and avoiding excessive alcohol or drug use can positively impact mental health.

3. Social Support: Building and maintaining strong social connections can provide a sense of belonging and support during challenging times. Connecting with friends, family, or support groups can help individuals feel understood and validated.

4. Stress Management: Developing effective stress management techniques, such as mindfulness meditation, deep breathing exercises, or engaging in activities that bring joy, can help individuals cope with stress and prevent it from negatively impacting mental health.

5. Seeking Professional Help: If individuals are experiencing persistent or severe mental health symptoms, it is essential to seek professional help. Mental health professionals, such as therapists or counselors, can provide guidance, support, and evidence-based treatments to address mental health concerns.

6.1.5 Breaking the Stigma

ONE OF THE SIGNIFICANT barriers to seeking help for mental health concerns is the stigma associated with mental illness. Stigma can lead to discrimination, isolation, and a reluctance to seek treatment. It is crucial to challenge and break down the stigma surrounding mental health by promoting open conversations, education, and understanding. By fostering a supportive and inclusive environment, individuals can feel more comfortable seeking help and support when needed.

6.1.6 Conclusion

UNDERSTANDING MENTAL health is essential for promoting overall well-being. By recognizing the importance of mental health, understanding common mental health conditions, and implementing strategies to promote mental well-being, individuals can take proactive steps towards leading a healthier and more fulfilling life. Remember, seeking help and support is a sign of strength, and everyone deserves to prioritize their mental health.

6.2 Stress Management Techniques

S tress is a common part of life that can have a significant impact on our overall well-being. It can affect us physically, mentally, and emotionally, and if left unmanaged, it can lead to a variety of health problems. Therefore, it is essential to develop effective stress management techniques to help us cope with and reduce the negative effects of stress.

6.2.1 Identifying Stressors

THE FIRST STEP IN MANAGING stress is to identify the sources of stress in our lives. These stressors can be external, such as work pressures, financial difficulties, or relationship problems. They can also be internal, such as negative self-talk, unrealistic expectations, or perfectionism. By recognizing and understanding our stressors, we can begin to develop strategies to address them effectively.

6.2.2 Relaxation Techniques

RELAXATION TECHNIQUES are an effective way to reduce stress and promote a sense of calm and well-being. These techniques can help activate the body's relaxation response, which counteracts the physiological effects of stress. Some popular relaxation techniques include the following:

• Deep breathing: Taking slow, deep breaths can help slow down the heart rate and promote relaxation. Practice deep breathing by inhaling deeply through your nose, holding your breath for a few seconds, and then exhaling slowly through your mouth.

• Progressive muscle relaxation: This technique involves tensing and then relaxing each muscle group in the body, starting from the toes and working your way up to the head. By consciously releasing tension in the muscles, you can promote a sense of relaxation and reduce stress.

• Meditation: Meditation involves focusing your attention and eliminating the stream of thoughts that may be causing stress. It can be as simple as sitting quietly and focusing on your breath or using guided meditation apps or videos.

• Yoga: Yoga combines physical postures, breathing exercises, and meditation to promote relaxation and reduce stress. Regular practice of yoga can help improve flexibility, strength, and overall well-being.

6.2.3 Time Management

POOR TIME MANAGEMENT can contribute to feelings of stress and overwhelm. By effectively managing our time, we can reduce stress and increase productivity. Here are some time management techniques to consider:

• Prioritize tasks: identify the most important tasks and tackle them first. This helps prevent procrastination and reduces the stress of feeling overwhelmed by a long to-do list.

• Break tasks into smaller steps: Breaking larger tasks into smaller, more manageable steps can make them feel less daunting and more achievable. This approach can help reduce stress and increase productivity.

• Set realistic goals: Setting realistic goals helps prevent feelings of failure and overwhelm. Break larger goals into smaller, achievable milestones, and celebrate your progress along the way.

• Delegate tasks: If possible, delegate tasks to others to lighten your workload. This can help reduce stress and free up time for more important or enjoyable activities.

6.2.4 Healthy Lifestyle Habits

MAINTAINING A HEALTHY lifestyle is crucial for managing stress. When we take care of our physical and mental well-being, we are better equipped to handle stress. Here are some healthy lifestyle habits that can help reduce stress:

• Regular exercise: Engaging in regular physical activity can help reduce stress and improve mood. Aim for at least 30 minutes of moderate-intensity exercise most days of the week.

• Healthy eating: A balanced diet rich in fruits, vegetables, whole grains, and lean proteins can provide the nutrients needed to support our physical and mental well-being. Avoid excessive caffeine, sugar, and processed foods, as they can contribute to feelings of stress and anxiety.

• Sufficient sleep: Getting enough quality sleep is essential for managing stress. Aim for 7-9 hours of sleep per night and establish a relaxing bedtime routine to promote better sleep.

• Limit alcohol and drug use: While alcohol and drugs may provide temporary relief from stress, they can ultimately contribute to feelings of anxiety and depression. Limiting or avoiding their use can help promote better mental and emotional well-being.

6.2.5 Mindfulness and Mind-Body Practices

MINDFULNESS AND MIND-body practices can help reduce stress and promote a sense of well-being. These practices involve focusing on the present moment and cultivating a non-judgmental awareness of our thoughts, feelings, and sensations. Some popular mindfulness and mind-body practices include:

• Mindful meditation: This practice involves focusing your attention on the present moment without judgment. It can be done sitting, lying down, or even while engaging in everyday activities like walking or eating.

• Tai chi: Tai chi is a gentle form of exercise that combines flowing movements with deep breathing and mental focus. It can help reduce stress, improve balance, and promote relaxation.

• Guided imagery: Guided imagery involves using your imagination to create a mental image of a peaceful, calming place. By visualizing this place, you can help reduce stress and promote relaxation.

• Journaling: Writing down your thoughts and feelings can help you gain insight into your stressors and emotions. It can also serve as a form of self-expression and stress relief.

6.2.6 Social Support

HAVING A STRONG SUPPORT system can significantly impact our ability to manage stress. Connecting with others and seeking support can provide a sense of belonging, understanding, and validation. Here are some ways to cultivate social support:

• Reach out to friends and family: Share your feelings and experiences with trusted friends and family members. They can provide emotional support and offer different perspectives on your stressors.

• Join support groups: Support groups provide a safe space to connect with others who may be experiencing similar challenges. They can offer valuable insights, coping strategies, and a sense of community.

• Seek professional help. If stress becomes overwhelming or begins to interfere with your daily life, consider seeking professional help. A therapist or counselor can provide guidance, support, and additional coping strategies.

By incorporating these stress management techniques into your daily life, you can effectively reduce stress and improve your overall well-being. Remember, managing stress is a lifelong journey, and it's essential to find what works best for you.

6.3 Building Resilience

Resilience is the ability to bounce back from adversity, cope with stress, and adapt to change. It is an essential skill for maintaining mental and emotional well-being. Building resilience can help you navigate life's challenges with greater ease and maintain a positive outlook even in the face of adversity. In this section, we will explore strategies and techniques to help you build resilience and enhance your overall well-being.

6.3.1 Understanding Resilience

RESILIENCE IS NOT SOMETHING we are born with; it is a skill that can be developed and strengthened over time. It involves developing a set of coping mechanisms and strategies that enable us to effectively deal with stress, setbacks, and difficult situations. Resilient individuals are better equipped to handle life's challenges and are more likely to experience positive outcomes in the face of adversity.

6.3.2 Building Resilience

BUILDING RESILIENCE requires a proactive approach and a commitment to personal growth. Here are some strategies to help you build resilience:

1. Cultivate a positive mindset.

MAINTAINING A POSITIVE mindset is crucial for building resilience. Focus on the positive aspects of your life and practice gratitude regularly. Surround yourself with positive and supportive people who uplift and inspire you. Engage in activities that bring you joy and help you maintain a positive outlook.

2. Develop strong social connections.

BUILDING STRONG SOCIAL connections is essential for resilience. Cultivate meaningful relationships with family, friends, and colleagues. Seek support from your loved ones during challenging times, and offer support to others when they need it. Having a strong support network can provide a sense of belonging and help you navigate difficult situations with greater ease.

3. Practice self-care.

TAKING CARE OF YOURSELF is vital for building resilience. Prioritize self-care activities that promote physical, mental, and emotional well-being. Engage in activities that help you relax and recharge, such as practicing mindfulness, engaging in hobbies, or spending time in nature. Make sure to get enough sleep, eat a balanced diet, and exercise regularly to support your overall well-being.

4. Develop problem-solving skills.

DEVELOPING PROBLEM-solving skills can enhance your resilience. Instead of dwelling on problems, focus on finding solutions. Break down challenges into smaller, manageable steps and brainstorm possible solutions. Seek advice and support from others when needed. Developing effective problem-solving skills can help you navigate difficult situations and find positive outcomes.

5. Practice stress management techniques.

STRESS IS A NATURAL part of life, but how we manage it can greatly impact our resilience. Explore different stress management techniques, such as deep breathing exercises, meditation, yoga, or journaling. Find what works best for you, and incorporate these techniques into your daily routine. Regularly practicing stress management techniques can help you build resilience and maintain a sense of calm during challenging times.

6. Embrace change and adaptability.

CHANGE IS INEVITABLE, and being able to adapt to new situations is a key aspect of resilience. Embrace change as an opportunity for growth and learning. Develop a flexible mindset and be open to new experiences. By embracing change and being adaptable, you can navigate life's challenges with greater ease and resilience.

6.3.3 Building Resilience in Children

BUILDING RESILIENCE in children is crucial for their overall well-being and future success. Here are some strategies to help children develop resilience:

1. Foster a supportive environment.

CREATE A SUPPORTIVE and nurturing environment for children to thrive. Encourage open communication, active listening, and empathy. Provide opportunities for children to express their emotions and validate their feelings. By fostering a supportive environment, children can develop a strong foundation for building resilience.

2. Encourage problem-solving skills.

TEACH CHILDREN PROBLEM-solving skills from an early age. Encourage them to think critically, explore different solutions, and make decisions. Provide guidance and support when needed, but also allow them to learn from their mistakes. By developing problem-solving skills, children can develop resilience and become more independent.

3. Teach coping mechanisms.

TEACH CHILDREN HEALTHY coping mechanisms to deal with stress and adversity. Encourage them to engage in activities they enjoy, such as art, music, or sports. Teach them relaxation techniques, such as deep breathing or visualization.

By teaching children healthy coping mechanisms, they can develop resilience and effectively manage stress throughout their lives.

4. Promote a growth mindset.

PROMOTE A GROWTH MINDSET in children by emphasizing the importance of effort, perseverance, and learning from mistakes. Encourage them to embrace challenges and view failures as opportunities for growth. By promoting a growth mindset, children can develop resilience and a positive attitude towards learning and personal development.

6.3.4 Seeking Help and Support

BUILDING RESILIENCE does not mean facing challenges alone. Seeking help and support is an important aspect of resilience. Reach out to trusted friends, family members, or professionals when you need assistance. Don't hesitate to seek therapy or counseling if you are struggling with your mental or emotional well-being. Remember, seeking help is a sign of strength, and it can greatly contribute to your overall resilience and well-being.

In conclusion, building resilience is a lifelong journey that requires commitment and practice. By cultivating a positive mindset, developing strong social connections, practicing self-care, and embracing change, you can enhance your resilience and navigate life's challenges with ease. Additionally, building resilience in children is crucial for their overall well-being and future success. By fostering a supportive environment, teaching problem-solving skills, and promoting a growth mindset, you can help children develop resilience from an early age. Remember, building resilience is a continuous process, and with time and practice, you can strengthen your ability to bounce back from adversity and thrive in all aspects of life.

6.4 Seeking Help and Support

Taking care of your mental and emotional well-being is just as important as taking care of your physical health. In times of difficulty or distress, seeking help and support can make a significant difference in your overall well-being. Whether you are facing a mental health challenge, dealing with stress, or simply need someone to talk to, there are various resources available to provide the support you need.

6.4.1 Recognizing the Need for Help

RECOGNIZING WHEN YOU need help is the first step towards seeking the support you require. It's essential to pay attention to your thoughts, feelings, and behaviors, as they can provide valuable insights into your mental and emotional state. If you notice any of the following signs persisting for an extended period, it may be time to seek help:

1. Persistent feelings of sadness, hopelessness, or emptiness.
2. loss of interest or pleasure in activities you once enjoyed.
3. changes in appetite or weight.
4. Difficulty sleeping or excessive sleeping
5. fatigue or lack of energy.

6. difficulty concentrating or making decisions.
7. thoughts of self-harm or suicide.
8. increased irritability or anger.
9. social withdrawal or isolation.
10. excessive worry or anxiety.

If you experience any of these symptoms, it's crucial to reach out to a healthcare professional or a mental health provider. They can help assess your situation, provide a diagnosis if necessary, and guide you towards appropriate treatment options.

6.4.2 Types of Help and Support

THERE ARE VARIOUS TYPES of help and support available for individuals seeking assistance with their mental and emotional well-being. Some of the most common options include:

6.4.2.1 Mental Health Professionals

MENTAL HEALTH PROFESSIONALS, such as psychologists, psychiatrists, and counselors, are trained to provide therapy and support for individuals experiencing mental health challenges. They can help you explore your thoughts and feelings, develop coping strategies, and work towards improving your overall well-being. These professionals can provide individual therapy, group therapy, or family therapy, depending on your specific needs.

6.4.2.2 Support Groups

SUPPORT GROUPS BRING together individuals who are facing similar challenges, providing a safe and supportive environment to share experiences, gain insights, and offer mutual support. These groups can be particularly helpful for individuals dealing with specific mental health conditions, such as depression, anxiety, or addiction. Support groups can be found in community centers, hospitals, or online platforms.

6.4.2.3 Helplines and Hotlines

HELPLINES AND HOTLINES offer immediate support and assistance to individuals in crisis or distress. These services are typically available 24/7 and provide a confidential and non-judgmental space for individuals to talk about their concerns. Helplines and hotlines are staffed by trained professionals who can offer guidance, crisis intervention, and referrals to appropriate resources.

6.4.2.4 Online Resources

THE INTERNET PROVIDES a wealth of resources for individuals seeking help and support for their mental and emotional well-being. Online platforms offer information, self-help tools, and virtual support communities where individuals can connect with others facing similar challenges. However, it's important to ensure that the online resources you access are reputable and trustworthy.

6.4.3 Overcoming Barriers to Seeking Help

SEEKING HELP AND SUPPORT for your mental and emotional well-being can sometimes be challenging due to various barriers. It's important to recognize and address these barriers to ensure you receive the assistance you need. Some common barriers include:

6.4.3.1 Stigma

STIGMA SURROUNDING mental health can prevent individuals from seeking help due to fear of judgment or discrimination. It's essential to remember that seeking help is a sign of strength, and mental health challenges are common and treatable. By challenging stigma and promoting open conversations about mental health, we can create a more supportive and understanding society.

6.4.3.2 Lack of Awareness

MANY INDIVIDUALS MAY not be aware of the available resources and support options for their mental and emotional well-being. It's important to educate yourself about the various services and organizations that can provide assistance. Talk to your healthcare provider, do research online, or reach out to local mental health organizations to learn about the resources available in your community.

6.4.3.3 Financial Constraints

FINANCIAL CONSTRAINTS can be a significant barrier to accessing mental health services. However, there are often low-cost or free options available, such as community mental health centers, sliding-scale fees, or government-funded programs. It's important to inquire about these options and explore all available avenues for support.

6.4.3.4 Cultural and Language Barriers

CULTURAL AND LANGUAGE barriers can make it challenging for individuals from diverse backgrounds to seek help. It's crucial to find mental health professionals or support groups that are culturally sensitive and can provide services in your preferred language. Many organizations offer multilingual services to ensure that individuals from different cultural backgrounds can access the support they need.

6.4.4 Building a Support Network

IN ADDITION TO PROFESSIONAL help, building a support network of friends, family, and loved ones can provide invaluable support for your mental and emotional well-being. Surrounding yourself with individuals who are understanding, empathetic, and supportive can make a significant difference in your overall well-being. Here are some tips for building a strong support network:

1. Communicate openly and honestly with your loved ones about your mental and emotional well-being.

2. Seek out individuals who are empathetic and non-judgmental.
3. Participate in activities and groups that align with your interests and values.
4. Join support groups or online communities where you can connect with individuals facing similar challenges.
5. Reach out to friends or family members when you need someone to talk to or lean on for support.
6. Consider seeking professional help to guide you in building a support network and developing coping strategies.

Remember, seeking help and support is a courageous step towards taking care of your mental and emotional well-being. By reaching out to the appropriate resources and building a strong support network, you can navigate life's challenges with resilience and find the support you need to thrive.

Healthy Relationships

7.1 Communication Skills

Effective communication is a fundamental aspect of building and maintaining healthy relationships. It is the key to expressing our thoughts, feelings, and needs, as well as understanding those of others. In the context of wellness, communication skills play a crucial role in promoting understanding, resolving conflicts, and fostering a supportive environment. This section will explore the importance of communication skills in various aspects of our lives and provide practical tips for improving them.

7.1.1 Active Listening

ACTIVE LISTENING IS a foundational communication skill that involves fully engaging with the speaker and demonstrating genuine interest in what they have to say. It goes beyond simply hearing the words and involves paying attention to non-verbal cues, such as body language and tone of voice. By practicing active listening, we can create a safe and supportive space for open and honest communication.

To become a better active listener, start by giving your full attention to the speaker. Avoid distractions and maintain eye contact. Show that you are listening by nodding, using verbal cues like "uh-huh" or "I see," and summarizing what the speaker has said. Avoid interrupting or jumping to conclusions. Instead, ask clarifying questions to ensure you have understood their message correctly.

7.1.2 Effective verbal communication

VERBAL COMMUNICATION is the primary means by which we express our thoughts, ideas, and emotions. Developing effective verbal communication skills can help us convey our message clearly and avoid misunderstandings. It involves using appropriate language, tone, and body language to effectively communicate our thoughts and feelings.

When engaging in verbal communication, it is important to choose your words carefully. Be mindful of the impact your words may have on others, and strive to use language that is respectful and inclusive. Pay attention to your tone of voice, as it can greatly influence how your message is received. Using a calm and assertive tone can help promote understanding and prevent conflicts.

Body language also plays a significant role in effective verbal communication. Maintain an open and relaxed posture, make eye contact, and use appropriate gestures to enhance your message. Avoid crossing your arms or displaying defensive body language, as it can create barriers to effective communication.

7.1.3 Non-Verbal Communication

NON-VERBAL COMMUNICATION refers to the messages we convey through facial expressions, gestures, and body language. It is an essential component of communication, as it can often convey more meaning than words alone. Being aware of and effectively using non-verbal cues can greatly enhance our ability to communicate with and understand others.

Facial expressions are a powerful form of non-verbal communication. A smile can convey warmth and friendliness, while a furrowed brow may indicate confusion or concern. Pay attention to the facial expressions of others, as they can provide valuable insights into their emotions and thoughts.

Gestures and body language also play a significant role in non-verbal communication. For example, nodding can indicate agreement or understanding, while crossing your arms may signal defensiveness or disagreement. Be mindful of the messages your body language is sending, and strive to use gestures that are open and welcoming.

7.1.4 Empathy and Understanding

EMPATHY IS THE ABILITY to understand and share the feelings of another person. It is a crucial skill in building and maintaining healthy relationships, as it allows us to connect with others on a deeper level. By practicing empathy, we can create an environment of understanding and support.

To cultivate empathy, try to put yourself in the other person's shoes and imagine how they might be feeling. Listen attentively to their concerns and validate their emotions. Avoid judgment or criticism, and instead offer support and understanding. By demonstrating empathy, you can foster trust and strengthen your relationships.

7.1.5 Assertive Communication

ASSERTIVE COMMUNICATION is a style of communication that allows individuals to express their thoughts, feelings, and needs in a respectful and confident manner. It involves clearly and directly stating your opinions and boundaries while considering the rights and feelings of others. Assertive communication can help prevent misunderstandings, resolve conflicts, and build healthier relationships.

To practice assertive communication, start by clearly stating your thoughts or needs using "I" statements. For example, instead of saying, "You never listen to me," try saying, "I feel unheard when I don't get a chance to express my thoughts." Use a calm and confident tone, maintain eye contact, and be open to listening to the other person's perspective. Remember to respect the boundaries and opinions of others while asserting your own.

7.1.6 Effective Feedback

PROVIDING AND RECEIVING feedback is an essential part of effective communication. Constructive feedback can help individuals grow and improve, while receiving feedback with an open mind can lead to personal development. When giving feedback, it is important to be specific, objective, and constructive. Focus on the behavior or action rather than the person, and offer suggestions for improvement. When receiving feedback, listen attentively, ask for clarification if needed, and be open to learning and growth.

7.1.7 Cultural Sensitivity

IN A DIVERSE AND MULTICULTURAL world, it is important to be culturally sensitive in our communication. Cultural sensitivity involves being aware of and respectful of the beliefs, values, and customs of different cultures. By practicing cultural sensitivity, we can avoid misunderstandings, promote inclusivity, and build stronger relationships.

To be culturally sensitive, take the time to educate yourself about different cultures and their communication norms. Avoid making assumptions or generalizations based on stereotypes. Instead, approach each individual with an open mind and a willingness to learn. Be respectful of cultural differences and adapt your communication style accordingly.

7.1.8 Conflict Resolution

CONFLICT IS A NATURAL part of any relationship, but how we handle it can greatly impact the outcome. Effective communication skills are essential to resolving conflicts in a healthy and constructive manner. When faced with a conflict, strive to understand the other person's perspective, express your own thoughts and feelings calmly and assertively, and work towards finding a mutually agreeable solution. Avoid blaming or attacking the other person, and instead focus on finding common ground and maintaining the relationship.

In conclusion, communication skills are vital for building and maintaining healthy relationships. By practicing active listening, effective verbal and non-verbal communication, empathy, assertiveness, and cultural sensitivity, we can enhance our ability to connect with others and promote understanding.

Conflict resolution and effective feedback are also important aspects of communication that can contribute to healthier relationships. By honing our communication skills, we can create a supportive and nurturing environment that fosters wellness and safety for ourselves and those around us.

7.2 Boundaries and Consent

Establishing and maintaining healthy boundaries is essential for fostering positive and respectful relationships. Boundaries help define what is acceptable and what is not, ensuring that individuals feel safe, respected, and valued. In addition to boundaries, consent plays a crucial role in healthy relationships, as it involves obtaining permission and respecting the autonomy of others. This section will explore the importance of boundaries and consent in various aspects of life and provide practical tips for establishing and maintaining them.

7.2.1 Understanding Boundaries

BOUNDARIES ARE PERSONAL limits that define the physical, emotional, and mental space we need to feel comfortable and safe. They serve as a protective barrier, preventing others from crossing into areas that make us feel vulnerable or violated. Boundaries can vary from person to person, and it is important to recognize and respect individual differences.

Setting personal boundaries

SETTING PERSONAL BOUNDARIES involves identifying and communicating your needs, desires, and limits to others. It is crucial to be aware of your own comfort levels and to assertively express them. This can be done by clearly communicating your boundaries, both verbally and non-verbally, and by consistently enforcing them. Remember that it is okay to say no and to prioritize your well-being.

Recognizing and Respecting Others' Boundaries

RESPECTING OTHERS' boundaries is equally important to maintaining healthy relationships. It involves being attentive to verbal and non-verbal cues and responding appropriately. It is essential to listen actively, show empathy, and avoid pressuring or manipulating others into crossing their boundaries. Respecting boundaries fosters trust, respect, and mutual understanding.

7.2.2 The Importance of Consent

CONSENT IS A FUNDAMENTAL aspect of healthy relationships and interactions. It involves obtaining explicit permission from all parties involved before engaging in any activity that may affect them physically, emotionally, or mentally. Consent should be enthusiastic, informed, and freely given, without any form of coercion or manipulation.

Consent in intimate relationships

IN INTIMATE RELATIONSHIPS, consent is crucial for ensuring that both partners feel comfortable and respected. It is essential to have open and honest communication about boundaries, desires, and limits. Consent should be ongoing and can be withdrawn at any time. It is important to remember that consent is not just about sexual activity but also extends to other aspects of the relationship, such as physical touch and personal boundaries.

Consent in Everyday Interactions

CONSENT IS NOT LIMITED to intimate relationships but applies to all interactions. It is important to seek consent before touching someone, sharing personal information, or engaging in activities that may affect others. Respecting personal boundaries and obtaining consent promotes a culture of respect, empathy, and understanding.

7.2.3 Establishing Boundaries and Consent in Different Settings

BOUNDARIES AND CONSENT are relevant in various settings, including personal relationships, the workplace, and social interactions. Here are some practical tips for establishing and maintaining boundaries and consent in different contexts:

Personal Relationships

- Communicate openly and honestly with your partner about your boundaries, desires, and limits.

- Respect your partner's boundaries and seek their consent before engaging in any activity.

- Regularly check in with each other to ensure that boundaries and consent are being respected.

- Seek professional help or counseling if you are struggling to establish or maintain healthy boundaries in your relationship.

Workplace

- Familiarize yourself with your organization's policies on boundaries and consent.

- Clearly communicate your boundaries and expectations to your colleagues and superiors.

- Report any instances of boundary violations or lack of consent to the appropriate authority.

- Advocate for a safe and respectful work environment for yourself and your colleagues.

Social Interactions

• Respect personal space and avoid touching others without their consent.

• Ask for permission before sharing personal information or discussing sensitive topics.

• Be mindful of others' boundaries and adjust your behavior accordingly.

• If someone expresses discomfort or withdraws consent, respect their decision and apologize if necessary.

7.2.4 Nurturing Healthy Boundaries and Consent

ESTABLISHING AND MAINTAINING healthy boundaries and consent is an ongoing process that requires self-awareness, communication, and practice. Here are some additional tips for nurturing healthy boundaries and consent:

• Reflect on your own needs, desires, and limits to gain a better understanding of your boundaries.

• Practice assertive communication to express your boundaries clearly and confidently.

• Surround yourself with individuals who respect and support your boundaries.

- Educate yourself about consent and stay informed about current discussions and developments.

- Regularly evaluate and reassess your boundaries to ensure they align with your evolving needs and values.

- Seek support from trusted friends, family members, or professionals if you are struggling with boundary-setting or consent-related issues.

Remember, boundaries and consent are essential for maintaining healthy and respectful relationships. By establishing and respecting boundaries and obtaining consent, you can create an environment that promotes trust, understanding, and well-being for yourself and those around you.

7.3 Conflict Resolution

Conflict is a natural part of human interaction. It can arise in various settings, including personal relationships, workplaces, and communities. While conflict can be uncomfortable and challenging, it also presents an opportunity for growth and resolution. In this section, we will explore effective strategies for resolving conflicts in a healthy and constructive manner.

7.3.1 Understanding Conflict

BEFORE DELVING INTO conflict resolution strategies, it is important to understand the nature of conflict. Conflict occurs when there is a disagreement or clash of interests between two or more parties. It can arise due to differences in values, beliefs, needs, or goals. Conflict can manifest in various forms, such as verbal arguments, passive-aggressive behavior, or even physical altercations.

It is crucial to recognize that conflict is not inherently negative. In fact, when managed effectively, conflict can lead to positive outcomes, such as improved communication, increased understanding, and strengthened relationships. However, if left unresolved, conflict can escalate and cause significant harm to individuals and relationships.

7.3.2 The Importance of Effective Conflict Resolution

RESOLVING CONFLICTS in a healthy and constructive manner is essential for maintaining positive relationships and promoting overall well-being. When conflicts are left unresolved, they can fester and create a toxic environment characterized by resentment, hostility, and emotional distress. On the other hand, addressing conflicts promptly and effectively can lead to resolution, reconciliation, and personal growth.

Effective conflict resolution has numerous benefits, including:

1. Improved Communication: Conflict resolution encourages open and honest communication, allowing individuals to express their thoughts, feelings, and concerns in a safe and respectful manner.

2. Enhanced Understanding: By actively listening and seeking to understand the perspectives of others, conflict resolution promotes empathy and fosters a deeper understanding of different viewpoints.

3. Strengthened Relationships: Resolving conflicts in a constructive manner can strengthen relationships by building trust, respect, and mutual understanding.

4. Reduced Stress: Unresolved conflicts can cause significant stress and emotional turmoil. By addressing conflicts and finding resolution, individuals can experience a sense of relief and reduced stress levels.

5. Personal Growth: Conflict resolution provides an

opportunity for personal growth and self-reflection. It allows individuals to develop problem-solving skills, emotional intelligence, and the ability to navigate challenging situations.

7.3.3 Strategies for Conflict Resolution

RESOLVING CONFLICTS requires a proactive and collaborative approach. Here are some effective strategies for conflict resolution:

1. Open and Respectful Communication: Effective communication is the foundation of conflict resolution. It is important to listen actively, express oneself clearly and respectfully, and avoid making assumptions or judgments. Use "I" statements to express your feelings and needs, and be open to hearing the perspectives of others.
2. Seek common ground: Look for areas of agreement and shared interests. Finding common ground can help build a foundation for resolving the conflict and finding mutually beneficial solutions.
3. Collaborative Problem-Solving: Instead of approaching conflict as a win-lose situation, strive for a win-win outcome. Collaborative problem-solving involves brainstorming solutions together and finding compromises that meet the needs of all parties involved.
4. Practice empathy: Put yourself in the shoes of the other person and try to understand their perspective. Empathy allows for greater understanding and can

help de-escalate conflicts.

5. Focus on the Issue, Not the Person: When resolving conflicts, it is important to separate the problem from the person. Avoid personal attacks or blame, and instead, focus on addressing the issue at hand.

6. Take a Break if Needed: If emotions are running high and the conflict becomes heated, it may be beneficial to take a break and revisit the discussion when everyone is calmer. This allows for a more productive and rational conversation.

7. Seek Mediation if Necessary: In some cases, conflicts may be complex or deeply rooted, making it challenging to find resolution on your own. In such situations, seeking the assistance of a neutral third party, such as a mediator or counselor, can be helpful in facilitating productive dialogue and finding a resolution.

7.3.4 Maintaining Healthy Relationships

CONFLICT RESOLUTION is not just about resolving immediate conflicts; it is also about building and maintaining healthy relationships in the long term. Here are some tips for fostering healthy relationships:

1. Practice active listening: Truly listen to others without interrupting or formulating responses in your mind. Show genuine interest and validate their feelings and experiences.

2. Respect Boundaries: Respect the boundaries and personal space of others. Be mindful of their comfort

levels and avoid crossing boundaries without consent.

3. Cultivate Empathy and Understanding: Seek to understand the perspectives and experiences of others. Empathy allows for greater compassion and connection.

4. Communicate Openly and Honestly: Foster an environment of open and honest communication. Encourage others to express their thoughts and feelings without fear of judgment or reprisal.

5. Show Appreciation and Gratitude: Express appreciation for the positive qualities and actions of others. Small gestures of gratitude can go a long way in strengthening relationships.

6. Resolve Conflicts Promptly: Address conflicts as they arise, rather than allowing them to fester and escalate. Prompt resolution prevents the accumulation of resentment and promotes healthier relationships.

7. Practice Forgiveness: Forgiveness is a powerful tool for healing and moving forward. Letting go of grudges and resentments allows for personal growth and the restoration of relationships.

Remember, conflict is a natural part of life, and resolving conflicts in a healthy and constructive manner is essential for personal well-being and the maintenance of positive relationships. By employing effective conflict resolution strategies and fostering healthy communication, you can navigate conflicts with grace and create a harmonious and supportive environment for yourself and those around you.

7.4 Building and Maintaining Relationships

Building and maintaining healthy relationships is an essential aspect of overall wellness. Strong and supportive relationships can have a positive impact on our mental, emotional, and physical well-being. They provide us with a sense of belonging, support, and love, which are crucial for our overall happiness and fulfillment. In this section, we will explore the importance of healthy relationships, effective communication skills, and strategies for resolving conflicts and maintaining strong connections with others.

7.4.1 The Importance of Healthy Relationships

HEALTHY RELATIONSHIPS are vital for our well-being, as they contribute to our overall happiness and quality of life. They provide us with emotional support, companionship, and a sense of belonging. Research has shown that individuals with strong social connections tend to have better mental health, lower levels of stress, and improved physical health.

Healthy relationships are built on trust, respect, and effective communication. They involve mutual understanding, empathy, and the ability to compromise. When we have healthy relationships, we feel safe, supported, and valued.

These relationships can be with family members, friends, romantic partners, or even colleagues.

7.4.2 Effective Communication Skills

EFFECTIVE COMMUNICATION is the foundation of any healthy relationship. It involves both expressing ourselves clearly and actively listening to others. Good communication allows us to understand each other's needs, feelings, and perspectives, leading to stronger connections and fewer misunderstandings.

To improve our communication skills, we can practice the following:

1. Active listening means paying full attention to the speaker, maintaining eye contact, and avoiding distractions. Reflecting on what the speaker is saying and asking clarifying questions will ensure understanding.

2. Non-verbal communication: being aware of our body language, facial expressions, and tone of voice. Non-verbal cues can convey emotions and intentions, so it's important to be mindful of how we present ourselves.

3. Empathy: putting ourselves in the other person's shoes and trying to understand their feelings and experiences. Showing empathy helps build trust and fosters a deeper connection.

4. Assertiveness: expressing our thoughts, feelings, and needs in a clear and respectful manner. Being assertive allows us to communicate our boundaries and expectations effectively.

5. Conflict Resolution: Addressing conflicts in a constructive and respectful way Listening to each other's perspectives, finding common ground, and working towards a mutually beneficial solution.

7.4.3 Strategies for Maintaining Relationships

MAINTAINING HEALTHY relationships requires effort and commitment from all parties involved. Here are some strategies to help nurture and strengthen your connections:

1. Quality Time: Spend quality time together, engaging in activities that you both enjoy. This can be as simple as having a meal together, going for a walk, or participating in a shared hobby.

2. Open and Honest Communication: Foster an environment of open and honest communication where both parties feel comfortable expressing their thoughts and feelings. Regularly check in with each other to ensure that you are on the same page.

3. Respect and Appreciation: Show respect and appreciation for one another. Acknowledge and celebrate each other's strengths and accomplishments. Express gratitude for the support and love you receive.

4. Boundaries: Establish and respect personal boundaries. Clearly communicate your needs and expectations, and be mindful of the other person's boundaries as well. This helps create a sense of safety and trust within the relationship.

5. Conflict Resolution: Address conflicts promptly and constructively. Listen to each other's perspectives,

validate each other's feelings, and work towards finding a resolution that satisfies both parties.

6. Support and Encouragement: Be supportive and encouraging of each other's goals and aspirations. Offer a listening ear, provide emotional support, and celebrate each other's successes.

7. Forgiveness: Practice forgiveness and let go of grudges. Holding onto past grievances can strain relationships, so it's important to forgive and move forward.

7.4.4 Seeking Help and Support

SOMETIMES, DESPITE our best efforts, relationships may face challenges that require outside help. It's important to recognize when professional support may be beneficial. Therapists, counselors, or relationship coaches can provide guidance and tools to navigate difficult situations and improve communication within the relationship.

Additionally, support groups or community organizations can offer a safe space to connect with others who may be experiencing similar relationship challenges. Sharing experiences and learning from others can provide valuable insights and support.

Remember, building and maintaining healthy relationships is an ongoing process that requires time, effort, and commitment from all parties involved. By prioritizing effective communication, mutual respect, and support, you can cultivate strong and fulfilling connections that contribute to your overall wellness and happiness.

Wellness for All Ages

8.1 Wellness in Childhood

C hildhood is a critical period for establishing healthy habits and promoting overall wellness. The choices made during these formative years can have a lasting impact on a child's physical, mental, and emotional well-being. In this section, we will explore the various aspects of wellness in childhood and provide practical tips for parents and caregivers to support their children's health and development.

8.1.1 Physical Health

PHYSICAL HEALTH IS a fundamental aspect of wellness in childhood. It encompasses various factors such as nutrition, exercise, and sleep. Ensuring that children receive a balanced diet rich in essential nutrients is crucial for their growth and development. Encourage the consumption of fruits, vegetables, whole grains, lean proteins, and dairy products to provide the necessary vitamins and minerals.

Regular physical activity is also vital for children's physical health. Encourage them to engage in age-appropriate activities such as running, jumping, swimming, or playing sports. Limit sedentary activities like watching television or playing video games, and promote outdoor play whenever possible.

Remember to prioritize safety by providing protective gear and supervising activities to prevent injuries.

Adequate sleep is essential for children's overall well-being. Establish a consistent bedtime routine and ensure that they get the recommended amount of sleep for their age. Create a calm and comfortable sleep environment, free from distractions such as electronic devices.

8.1.2 Mental and Emotional Well-Being

PROMOTING MENTAL AND emotional well-being in childhood is crucial for building resilience and preventing mental health issues later in life. Encourage open communication and create a supportive and nurturing environment where children feel comfortable expressing their thoughts and emotions. Listen actively and validate their feelings, helping them develop healthy coping mechanisms.

Teach children stress management techniques such as deep breathing exercises, mindfulness, and engaging in activities they enjoy. Encourage them to participate in creative outlets like drawing, painting, or playing musical instruments, which can serve as effective outlets for self-expression and emotional release.

Building strong social connections is also essential for children's mental and emotional well-being. Encourage them to develop friendships, participate in group activities, and engage in positive social interactions. Teach them empathy, kindness, and respect for others, fostering healthy relationships and a sense of belonging.

8.1.3 Intellectual Development

INTELLECTUAL DEVELOPMENT plays a significant role in a child's overall wellness. Stimulate their curiosity and love for learning by providing age-appropriate educational materials and engaging in activities that promote cognitive development. Read to them regularly, and encourage independent reading as they grow older. Engage in educational games, puzzles, and activities that challenge their problem-solving skills and critical thinking abilities.

Limit screen time and ensure that the content they consume is educational and age-appropriate. Encourage them to explore their interests and pursue hobbies that stimulate their intellectual growth. Support their education by actively engaging with their schoolwork and providing a conducive environment for learning.

8.1.4 Social Skills and Emotional Intelligence

DEVELOPING SOCIAL SKILLS and emotional intelligence is crucial for children's overall well-being and future success. Teach them effective communication skills, including active listening, expressing themselves clearly, and resolving conflicts peacefully. Encourage them to understand and respect others' boundaries and consent, promoting healthy relationships and empathy.

Provide opportunities for children to interact with peers and engage in cooperative activities that foster teamwork and collaboration. Teach them problem-solving skills and encourage them to find solutions independently, promoting their autonomy and self-confidence.

8.1.5 Safety and Injury Prevention

ENSURING THE SAFETY of children is paramount for their well-being. Create a safe environment by childproofing the home, removing potential hazards, and securing dangerous substances. Teach children about safety rules, such as crossing the road, using seat belts, and wearing helmets when riding bicycles or participating in sports.

Educate children about personal safety, including stranger danger and appropriate boundaries. Teach them how to recognize and respond to emergencies, including dialing emergency services. Regularly review safety measures and update children on any changes or new information.

8.1.6 Regular Health Check-ups and Immunizations

REGULAR HEALTH CHECK-ups and immunizations are essential for maintaining children's wellness. Schedule routine visits with a pediatrician to monitor their growth and development, address any concerns, and receive necessary vaccinations. Stay informed about the recommended immunization schedule and ensure that children receive all the required vaccines to protect against preventable diseases.

By prioritizing wellness in childhood, parents and caregivers can lay a strong foundation for their children's future health and well-being. By promoting physical health, supporting mental and emotional well-being, fostering intellectual development, and ensuring safety, children can thrive and reach their full potential. Remember that each child is unique, and it is essential to tailor strategies to their individual needs and preferences.

8.2 Wellness in Adolescence

Adolescence is a critical period of growth and development, both physically and emotionally. It is a time of transition from childhood to adulthood, marked by significant changes in the body, brain, and social relationships. During this stage, young people experience rapid physical growth, hormonal changes, and the development of their identity and independence. It is essential to prioritize wellness during adolescence to support healthy development and lay the foundation for a lifetime of well-being.

8.2.1 Physical Health

PHYSICAL HEALTH IS a fundamental aspect of wellness in adolescence. It is crucial to maintain a healthy lifestyle by engaging in regular physical activity, eating a balanced diet, and getting enough sleep. Regular exercise not only helps to maintain a healthy weight but also improves cardiovascular health, strengthens bones and muscles, and boosts mood and mental well-being. Encourage adolescents to participate in activities they enjoy, such as sports, dancing, or hiking, to make exercise a fun and sustainable habit.

A nutritious diet is essential for supporting growth and development during adolescence. Encourage adolescents to consume a variety of fruits, vegetables, whole grains, lean proteins, and low-fat dairy products. Limit the intake of sugary drinks, processed foods, and snacks high in saturated fats and added sugars. It is also important to promote healthy eating habits, such as eating regular meals, avoiding skipping breakfast, and practicing mindful eating.

Adequate sleep is crucial for physical and mental well-being during adolescence. Encourage adolescents to establish a consistent sleep schedule and prioritize getting the recommended 8–10 hours of sleep per night. Limiting screen time before bed, creating a relaxing bedtime routine, and ensuring a comfortable sleep environment can help promote healthy sleep habits.

8.2.2 Emotional Well-Being

ADOLESCENCE IS A TIME of emotional growth and self-discovery. It is common for adolescents to experience a range of emotions, including excitement, joy, stress, and sadness. Promoting emotional well-being involves helping adolescents develop healthy coping mechanisms, manage stress, and build resilience.

Encourage open and honest communication with adolescents, creating a safe space for them to express their feelings and concerns. Teach them healthy ways to cope with stress, such as deep breathing exercises, engaging in hobbies or activities they enjoy, and seeking support from trusted friends, family members, or professionals when needed.

Building resilience is essential for navigating the challenges and setbacks that may arise during adolescence. Encourage adolescents to develop problem-solving skills, set realistic goals, and practice self-care. Encourage them to engage in activities that promote self-expression and self-reflection, such as journaling, art, or mindfulness exercises.

8.2.3 Social Relationships

SOCIAL RELATIONSHIPS play a significant role in adolescent wellness. Adolescents are navigating the complexities of friendships, romantic relationships, and family dynamics. It is important to support healthy relationships and provide guidance on setting boundaries, practicing consent, and resolving conflicts.

Encourage adolescents to develop effective communication skills, including active listening, expressing themselves assertively, and respecting others' perspectives. Teach them about the importance of consent and the boundaries that should be respected in all relationships. Help them understand the value of healthy relationships built on trust, respect, and mutual support.

8.2.4 Mental Health

ADOLESCENCE IS A TIME when mental health issues may emerge or become more pronounced. It is crucial to prioritize mental health and provide support for adolescents who may be experiencing challenges such as anxiety, depression, or stress.

Promote mental well-being by encouraging adolescents to engage in activities that promote relaxation and stress reduction, such as practicing mindfulness, engaging in hobbies, or spending time in nature. Teach them to recognize the signs of mental health issues in themselves and others and to seek help when needed. Provide information about available mental health resources, such as school counselors, therapists, or helplines.

8.2.5 Healthy Habits for Life

ADOLESCENCE IS A CRITICAL period for establishing healthy habits that can last a lifetime. Encourage adolescents to take responsibility for their well-being by making informed choices about their health and safety. Provide them with the knowledge and skills to navigate challenges, make healthy decisions, and advocate for their own well-being.

By prioritizing wellness in adolescence, young people can develop the resilience, skills, and habits necessary to lead healthy and fulfilling lives. Empower them to take control of their well-being and support them in their journey towards optimal health and safety.

8.3 Wellness in Adulthood

Adulthood is a significant phase in life where individuals experience various changes and responsibilities. It is a time when personal well-being becomes even more crucial as we navigate through the challenges and demands of work, relationships, and family life. In this section, we will explore the key aspects of wellness in adulthood and provide practical tips to help you maintain a healthy and balanced lifestyle.

8.3.1 Physical Health

PHYSICAL HEALTH IS the foundation of overall well-being, and it becomes increasingly important as we age. In adulthood, it is essential to prioritize regular exercise, healthy eating habits, and preventive healthcare measures. Engaging in regular physical activity not only helps maintain a healthy weight but also improves cardiovascular health, strengthens muscles and bones, and boosts mood and energy levels. Aim for at least 150 minutes of moderate-intensity aerobic activity or 75 minutes of vigorous-intensity aerobic activity per week, along with muscle-strengthening activities twice a week.

A well-balanced diet is crucial for maintaining optimal health in adulthood. Focus on consuming a variety of nutrient-dense foods, including fruits, vegetables, whole grains, lean proteins, and healthy fats. Limit the intake of processed foods, sugary beverages, and excessive salt. Stay hydrated by drinking an adequate amount of water throughout the day.

Regular check-ups and screenings are vital for the early detection and prevention of potential health issues. Schedule routine visits with your healthcare provider to monitor your blood pressure, cholesterol levels, and other key health indicators. Stay up-to-date with vaccinations and immunizations recommended for adults, such as influenza, tetanus, and shingles vaccines.

8.3.2 Mental and Emotional Well-Being

MAINTAINING GOOD MENTAL and emotional well-being is equally important in adulthood. As we face various responsibilities and challenges, it is essential to prioritize self-care and stress management. Practice stress-reducing techniques such as deep breathing exercises, meditation, and mindfulness to promote relaxation and reduce anxiety.

Building resilience is crucial for navigating the ups and downs of life. Cultivate a positive mindset, develop problem-solving skills, and seek support from friends, family, or a mental health professional when needed. Engage in activities that bring you joy and fulfillment, whether it's pursuing a hobby, spending time in nature, or practicing gratitude.

8.3.3 Healthy Relationships

NURTURING HEALTHY RELATIONSHIPS is a vital aspect of well-being in adulthood. Cultivate open and effective communication skills to express your needs, thoughts, and emotions clearly. Practice active listening and empathy to foster understanding and connection with others.

Establishing and maintaining boundaries is essential for healthy relationships. Clearly define your limits and communicate them assertively. Respect the boundaries of others and be mindful of their needs and comfort levels.

Conflict resolution skills are valuable in maintaining harmonious relationships. Learn effective strategies for resolving conflicts, such as active listening, compromise, and finding common ground. Seek professional help if needed to navigate challenging relationship dynamics.

Building and maintaining relationships requires effort and investment. Prioritize spending quality time with loved ones, whether it's through shared activities, meaningful conversations, or simply being present. Surround yourself with positive and supportive individuals who uplift and inspire you.

8.3.4 Career and Financial Wellness

CAREER SATISFACTION and financial stability play a significant role in overall well-being during adulthood. Strive for a career that aligns with your passions and values, as this can contribute to a sense of purpose and fulfillment. Continuously invest in your professional development through learning opportunities, networking, and skill-building.

Financial wellness involves managing your finances responsibly and planning for the future. Create a budget, track your expenses, and save for emergencies and long-term goals. Seek professional advice if needed to ensure you are making informed decisions about investments, retirement planning, and debt management.

8.3.5 Personal Growth and Fulfillment

PERSONAL GROWTH AND fulfillment are essential components of wellness in adulthood. Continuously seek opportunities for self-improvement and personal development. Set goals that align with your values and aspirations, and take steps towards achieving them.

Engage in activities that bring you joy, fulfillment, and a sense of purpose. Explore new hobbies, pursue creative outlets, or volunteer for causes that resonate with you. Cultivate a positive mindset and practice self-compassion, celebrating your achievements and learning from setbacks.

Remember to prioritize self-care and make time for activities that recharge and rejuvenate you. This may include practicing mindfulness, engaging in hobbies, spending time in nature, or seeking support from loved ones.

In conclusion, wellness in adulthood encompasses various aspects of physical, mental, and emotional well-being. By prioritizing regular exercise, healthy eating, preventive healthcare, and stress management, you can maintain optimal physical health. Nurturing healthy relationships, establishing boundaries, and developing effective communication and conflict resolution skills contribute to emotional well-being. Career satisfaction, financial stability, personal growth, and fulfillment are also crucial for overall wellness in adulthood. By incorporating these practices into your daily life, you can lead a balanced, fulfilling, and healthy adulthood.

8.4 Wellness in Older Adults

As we age, it becomes increasingly important to prioritize our wellness and safety. Older adults face unique challenges and considerations when it comes to maintaining their health and well-being. In this section, we will explore the specific aspects of wellness that are important for older adults and provide practical tips and strategies for promoting a healthy and fulfilling life in the golden years.

8.4.1 Physical Health

PHYSICAL HEALTH IS a crucial component of overall wellness, and it becomes even more important as we age. Older adults may experience changes in their bodies that can impact their mobility, strength, and overall physical well-being. However, with the right approach, it is possible to maintain and even improve physical health in later life.

Regular exercise is key to promoting physical health in older adults. Engaging in activities such as walking, swimming, or yoga can help improve strength, flexibility, and balance. It is important to choose exercises that are appropriate for your fitness level and take into account any existing health conditions or limitations. Consulting with a healthcare professional or a certified fitness instructor can help you develop a safe and effective exercise routine.

In addition to exercise, maintaining a healthy diet is essential for older adults. A well-balanced diet that includes a variety of fruits, vegetables, whole grains, lean proteins, and healthy fats can provide the necessary nutrients to support overall health. It is also important to stay hydrated and limit the consumption of processed foods, sugary drinks, and excessive amounts of salt.

Regular check-ups with healthcare professionals are crucial for older adults to monitor their physical health. These check-ups can help identify any potential health issues early on and allow for timely intervention. It is important to follow recommended screenings and preventive measures, such as mammograms, colonoscopies, and vaccinations, to maintain optimal health.

8.4.2 Mental and Emotional Well-Being

MENTAL AND EMOTIONAL well-being are equally important for older adults as physical health. Aging can bring about various life changes and challenges that may impact mental health. It is important to prioritize self-care and seek support when needed to maintain a positive outlook and emotional well-being.

Engaging in activities that promote mental stimulation and cognitive function is beneficial for older adults. Activities such as reading, puzzles, learning new skills, and socializing can help keep the mind sharp and improve overall mental well-being. It is also important to maintain social connections and engage in meaningful relationships, as social isolation can have a negative impact on mental health.

Managing stress is crucial for older adults, as chronic stress can contribute to various health issues. Practicing stress management techniques such as deep breathing exercises, meditation, and engaging in hobbies or activities that bring joy and relaxation can help reduce stress levels. Seeking professional help, such as therapy or counseling, can also be beneficial for managing stress and addressing any underlying mental health concerns.

8.4.3 Safety and Independence

MAINTAINING SAFETY and independence is a top priority for older adults. Taking proactive measures to create a safe environment can help prevent accidents and injuries. Simple modifications to the home, such as installing grab bars in the bathroom, removing tripping hazards, and ensuring proper lighting, can significantly reduce the risk of falls.

Regularly reviewing and updating medications is important for older adults to prevent adverse drug interactions and ensure the correct dosage. It is advisable to keep an updated list of medications and share it with healthcare professionals to avoid any potential complications.

Having a plan in place for emergencies is crucial for older adults. This includes having emergency contact information readily available, knowing how to access medical assistance, and having a support system in place. It is also important to consider options for long-term care and to have conversations with loved ones about preferences and wishes for future care.

8.4.4 Seeking Support and Resources

NAVIGATING THE COMPLEXITIES of aging can be challenging, but there are numerous resources and support systems available to older adults. It is important to be proactive in seeking out these resources and utilizing the support that is available.

Local community centers, senior centers, and organizations dedicated to older adults often offer a wide range of programs and services. These can include exercise classes, educational workshops, social activities, and support groups. Engaging in these activities can provide opportunities for socialization, learning, and support.

Family and friends can also be a valuable source of support for older adults. Maintaining open lines of communication and reaching out for help when needed is important. Additionally, healthcare professionals, such as doctors, nurses, and therapists, can provide guidance and support in managing health concerns and navigating the aging process.

In conclusion, wellness in older adults encompasses physical, mental, and emotional well-being, as well as safety and independence. By prioritizing regular exercise, maintaining a healthy diet, seeking support, and creating a safe environment, older adults can enjoy a fulfilling and healthy life. It is important to be proactive in taking care of one's health and to utilize the resources and support systems available. Aging is a natural part of life, and with the right approach, it can be a time of growth, fulfillment, and well-being.

Also by imed el arbi

Metamorphosis Mindset: Transforming Your Life, One Thought at a Time
Life Mastery: a Toolkit for Success
Your Hidden Power of Mind: Unleashing Your Full Potential
Rise to Radiance
Realize Your Ultimate Potential
Revitalize Your Reality: The Art of Life Transformation
Transforming Within: A Path to Personal Evolution

YouTube Secrets
YouTube Secrets: Build a Successful Channel in 5 Days
YouTube Secrets: Build a Successful Channel with Artificial Intelligence
YouTube Secrets: the Ultimate Guide to Creating Popular and Successful Content

Standalone
The Magical Woodland Adventure

The Money Mindset Makeover: Unleashing True Financial
Potential
Digital Deception: A Detective Jane Miller Mystery
The Enigma of Slytherin's Legacy
Bound by Love and Betrayal: an Immigrant's Journey
Tesla's 369 Revelation: A Journey to Spiritual Power
Silencing the Inner Critic: Unleashing Your True Potential
Smoke-Free Success: a Path to Health and Wealth
Navigating Success: 7 Principles of High Achievers
Charm 101: the Art of Wooing Women
Motivate Your Mind: Mastering Motivation for Success
Enchanting Cities: Exploring the World's Urban Treasures
How to Build a Successful Career in the Gig Economy
Mindful Living in the Digital Era
Raising Resilient Kids: a Mindful Guide to Parenting
The Compassionate Self: Cultivating Kindness Within
The Science of Happiness: The Pursuit of Joy
Freelance Writing Success: Launch, Grow, and Scale Your
Career
Emotional Well-being: A Guide to Mental Health
HABITS RICH PEOPLE WON'T TELL YOU
Rich Habits, Rich Life: Mastering the Art of Wealth Building
Rising Horizons: Accelerating Business Development
The Lost City of Mythica: Uncovering Mythica's Secret
Generational Harmony: Winning Through Diversity
Alchemy of the Soul: A Roadmap to Life Transformation
Rise Strong: Embracing Resilience and Renewal
AI Riches: Unleashing the Profit Potential of Artificial
Intelligence
Building Your Online Store with WooCommerce
Online Entrepreneurship: Success Roadmap

Shopify Mastery: The Ultimate Guide to E-commerce Success
Thriving Freelance: A Guide to Writing on Your Own Terms
Habit Mastery: A Simple Guide to Building Good Habits and Stopping Negative Ones
Reading Between the Gestures: A Brief Manual on Body Language
Bridges Across Cultures: Short story collection
Harmony in the Digital Jungle: Unveiling the Secrets of Home-Based Success
Cultivating Creativity: Fostering Innovation in Educational Settings
Gamification in Education: Leveling Up Learning Experiences
Mathematical Mastery: Unleashing the Power of Teaching
Smart Classrooms, Smarter Students: Navigating the AI Revolution in Education
Adapting Thinking Classrooms: Guide for Inclusive Education.
Flexible Thinking Classrooms: Enhancing Learning in Various Environments
Navigating the Pedagogical Landscape: Strategies for 21st-Century Educators
Revolutionary Teaching: Unleashing the Power of Pedagogy
Teaching for Tomorrow: Bridging Theory and Practice
Student-Centered Pedagogy for Lifelong Success
Differential pedagogy : How to distinguish individual differences between learners ?
Eternal Vitality: Mastering the Art of Longevity
Ink and Heart: A Guide to Transformative Teaching
The New Rich: Redefining Work-Life Balance in the Modern Age
Wellness and Safety: A Guide to Health and Care

Milton Keynes UK
Ingram Content Group UK Ltd.
UKHW010836071223
433828UK00001B/22

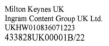

9 798215 952214